Evidence-Based Decisionmaking for Community Health Programs

Catherine A. Jackson
Kathryn Pitkin
Raynard Kington

Prepared for the
Main Line Health System

RAND

RA
425
J32
1998

MAR 24 1998

PREFACE

This report explores how scientific evidence can help inform decisions about the funding and evaluation of community-based health interventions. It should interest persons and organizations that fund or implement community-based health programs, particularly those who want to understand more about program evaluation and how evaluative data can be used to make program decisions.

The research reported here arose from discussions between RAND staff and Arnold Tiemeyer, Vice President of Community Services for Main Line Health System in Philadelphia, Pennsylvania, about how today's health care systems make decisions about community-based health interventions. A recurrent question was whether foundations and other funders used evidence-based approaches to decide which programs to fund and whether they routinely assessed the success of community-based programs. This study was supported by the Main Line Health System with additional funding from The Robert Wood Johnson Foundation.

This report was written while Raynard Kington was a Senior Natural Scientist at RAND.

CONTENTS

Preface iii
Summary vii
Acknowledgments xiii

Chapter One
    INTRODUCTION 1

Chapter Two
    AN EVIDENCE-BASED APPROACH TO
    DECISIONMAKING FOR COMMUNITY HEALTH
    INTERVENTIONS 3

Chapter Three
    IS THERE ENOUGH EVIDENCE TO SUPPORT AN
    EVIDENCE-BASED APPROACH? 9
    Method 10
    Findings 12
    Discussion 15
        Scientific Rigor of Evaluation and Effectiveness
            Research 15
        Outcome Measures and Comparisons Across Potential
            Interventions 16
        Access to Information on Implementation 17

Chapter Four
    THE VIEW FROM HEALTH CARE SYSTEMS AND
    FUNDERS: FOCUS GROUPS 19
    Method 19
    Findings 20

       What Drives Funding Priorities 21
       How Organizations Make Funding Decisions 22
       Program Evaluation 24
       Information Needed 27
   Summary 27

Chapter Five
THE VIEW FROM HEALTH CARE SYSTEMS AND
FUNDERS: TELEPHONE INTERVIEWS 29
   Method 29
   Findings 31
       Types of Programs Funded 31
       How Organizations Make Funding Decisions 32
       Program Evaluation 34
       Information Needed 36
   Summary 38

Chapter Six
TOWARD AN EVIDENCE-BASED APPROACH TO
COMMUNITY HEALTH INTERVENTIONS 41
   Health Care Systems 44
   Private Funders 45

Appendix
   A. Literature Identified 47
   B. Focus Group Protocol: Funders 71
   C. Telephone Interviews: Suggested Questions for Health
      Systems 77

References 81

SUMMARY

Medical practice in the United States has gravitated over the past generation toward an "evidence-based" approach. In this approach, data from randomized clinical trials and other scientific sources inform decisions made by clinicians caring for the health of individual patients. Attempts are made to evaluate the success of these decisions by monitoring patient health outcomes. The evidence-based approach represents a break from a history of physician decision-making overly influenced by tradition, protocol, and habit.

The move to evidence-based medicine has partly been driven by a growing desire for better patient care and greater efficiency. Yet, though such aims would appear to be important for all aspects of health care, less attention has been paid to the evidence-based approach outside hospitals, clinics, and doctor's offices. And it is outside those facilities—in schools, churches, senior centers, and elsewhere in the community—that health care providers and others are beginning to carry out many important health promotion and disease and injury prevention activities. Could an evidence-based approach inform decisions made about such community-level health programs? Could it help in testing the effectiveness of, and allocating funds among, such programs as parenting classes, anti-smoking advertisements, and mammography promotion?

We sought answers to these questions. In particular, we wanted to know whether evidence regarding the cost and effectiveness of community health programs was even available, and, if so, how health care organizations and foundations funding community programs used that evidence. To seek answers, we conducted a review of the public health and medical literature for studies on community health programs and interviewed decisionmakers at health care organizations and foundations, both collectively in focus groups and individually by telephone.

DEFINITION AND MOTIVATION

Before we report our findings, it may be helpful to say what we mean by an evidence-based approach in the community context and why such an approach may be a wise one. At the community level, the evidence-based approach may be understood as one in which

- decisions about community health interventions are informed by the best evidence available about individual behavior, population characteristics, and strategies to promote health;
- the use of such information in decisionmaking is mediated by specific community characteristics, goals, resources, and even values; and
- the effectiveness and costs of the resulting interventions are continuously evaluated.

The argument in favor of such an approach is straightforward. As the organization of medical practice shifts increasingly to managed care, health care systems are thinking of their mission more in terms of satisfying the needs of populations instead of individuals. Furthermore, health promotion and disease prevention actions taken in community settings may prove more cost-effective than therapeutic actions taken later in clinical settings. But some basis is required for deciding in which community health interventions to invest limited resources. Foundations may also find an evidence-based approach useful as they seek to close what are likely to be growing gaps in health and access to health care, especially for vulnerable populations such as immigrants. The evidence-based approach provides an aid to decisionmaking tailored to realizing the greatest gain per dollar spent.

THE AVAILABLE EVIDENCE

The evidence-based approach begins, of course, with evidence, and the results of our literature search implied an important obstacle to implementing that approach at the community level: There is little evidence available. We searched two commercial databases for articles published since 1980. After eliminating articles on clinical interventions, our search yielded only 30 articles we considered relevant to the application of an evidence-based model in a community context. Of those, about half were in school settings. Most used quasi-experimental assessment methods. The choice of outcome measures varied considerably, and relatively few studies discussed in detail the meaning of the magnitude of the difference in outcome measures between the intervention and the control. Only two of the papers clearly concluded that the intervention did not have any of the desired effects. This suggests that journals or investigators are selecting against the publication of negative results, information which is important for the evidence-based approach. Only one of the papers included an analysis of costs, and that was relatively crude. And many of the evaluations did not contain enough information on the nature of the intervention to support inferences regarding costs.

These problems—lack of information on negative results and costs—are not unique to community interventions. Clinical interventions face similar problems. The literature thus does not generally allow the comparison of interventions in terms of benefits derived per dollar spent. For example, if a community-based organization wanted to choose between a school-based intervention targeting drug abuse and a community-wide intervention to prevent HIV, the literature would not provide much guidance.

CURRENT DECISIONMAKING PRACTICES AND NEEDS

Through the interviews, conducted simultaneously with the literature review, we hoped to learn more about the feasibility of implementing an evidence-based approach in the community context. We also sought to learn what drives funding decisions, how funded programs are evaluated, and what types of information would be useful in performing evaluations. We ran four focus groups—one in Los Angeles and three in Philadelphia—each with three or four individuals representing foundation program staff, foundation board members, and staff of foundation-funded, community-based programs. We also conducted nine telephone interviews—six with foundation representatives and three with representatives of health care organizations in different parts of the country.

Foundation staff generally defined their mission expansively as doing good in the community, often for one group or another, e.g., the disadvantaged, women, children, and the elderly. Often, staff identified what "good" was through intuition or gut reaction to observed conditions. Scientific evidence of likely program effectiveness did not play a large role. The general consensus was that very few proposals included such evidence that the proposed program would achieve its stated goals. "Evidence" of potential success often took the form of testimonials regarding organizational credibility solicited from an informal network of third parties. In fact, almost all focus group participants acknowledged a reluctance to make funding decisions solely on information about a given intervention's effectiveness. They held it necessary to account for community- and organization-specific information. Furthermore, several organizations wanted to take risks and expected that an appreciable fraction of funded activities would fail to achieve their goals; evidence suggesting predictable success would thus be less interesting to such organizations.

Although foundations typically required evaluation plans from those submitting proposals, the quality of those plans was quite variable. Formal evaluations that could yield scientifically sound conclusions were uncommon. These were usually believed to be a drain on the resources of both the foundation and the proposer. Few community organizations have the resources to monitor outcomes over time. Therefore, often the only outcome measure available to funders was the number of individuals served.

All those we interviewed expressed an interest in obtaining more information as to the effectiveness of community-based health interventions. Some mentioned the potential for collaboration with universities, but none seemed ready to abandon judgment and "street sense" as important elements in making funding decisions.

TOWARD AN EVIDENCE-BASED APPROACH

In the clinical context, the evolution of evidence-based medical practice has been facilitated by several factors—wide acceptance of randomized clinical trials, unexplained variations in procedure use that suggested some utilization was unnecessary, and growing pressure to control costs. In contrast, the road to evidence-based decisionmaking on community health interventions is strewn with impediments, and it is important to recognize these:

- The professional community has not come to a consensus on a "gold standard" for ranking the strength of scientific evidence for community-based interventions even though social research textbooks and authors have outlined the relative strengths and weaknesses of various study designs. This is partly because experimental designs are inordinately expensive to implement in community settings.

- There are few comprehensive data on the universe of community health programs, for example, rates of participation, funding levels, variation across communities, costs, and outcomes or effects. Thus, there is insufficient basis for claims of inefficiency that might motivate more rigorous funding decisions.

- Moreover, funders of community interventions are often not facing a specific health problem to be solved, as a clinician is, but responding to a more generalized desire to do good for the community.

- No one organization pays the costs for, and reaps the benefits from, a community health intervention. Funding and implementation decisions involve public health departments, managed care providers, foundations, and community-based organizations. Furthermore, one organization may pay for an intervention whose benefits are realized only much later when an individual's care is the financial responsibility of another organization.

Notwithstanding these difficulties, there are steps that health care organizations and private funders such as foundations can take to promote evidence-based decisionmaking on community health interventions. Health care organizations could:

- allocate a portion of their budget for community-based interventions to those for which there is quantitative evidence of effectiveness;
- work with community-based organizations and public health departments to coordinate community-wide strategies for the implementation and evaluation of health care interventions;
- partner with each other and with academic and research institutions to promote rigorous evaluations of interventions;
- start collecting data on the costs of all interventions; and
- incorporate into requests for external funds as much as feasible the best evidence that proposed interventions will work.

Private funders such as foundations could:

- fund a consortium to establish standards of evidence (e.g., study designs, outcome measures, and minimum data needs) regarding the effectiveness and costs of community-based health interventions;
- fund costs of evaluation, especially the collection of meaningful cost data;
- promote the collection of information describing and monitoring the full range of community health interventions now funded;
- promote the establishment of centralized sources of information on community-based interventions and the establishment of regional coalitions that can provide technical assistance to organizations wishing to undertake more rigorous evaluations;
- fund research to assess the economic effect of community-based interventions for managed care organizations;
- provide greater incentives for organizations to be open in disseminating evidence about interventions that do not achieve their goals; and
- fund workshops and conferences and write editorials promoting open discussion of the potential of evidence-based decisionmaking to improve the effectiveness and efficiency of community-based interventions.

ACKNOWLEDGMENTS

This project owes its existence to the interest of Arnold Tiemeyer of Main Line Health System. We are grateful for his insight, his help in acquiring funding from The Robert Wood Johnson Foundation, and his participation in the focus groups.

We have also benefited from the assistance of our colleagues at RAND. M. Audrey Burnam offered helpful comments in her review of the report, and James Chiesa enhanced the clarity of the report. Finally, we thank our research assistant, Deirdra Forte, who was principally responsible for reading over 100 articles identified as potentially relevant in our literature review and for the initial judgments as to whether they could support an evidence-based approach.

Many individuals, listed below, generously contributed their time and thoughts to this project. We appreciate their participation. Their remarks have greatly contributed to our enriched understanding of foundations' decisionmaking processes.

Catherine Clark, M.D., Main Line Health System Board, Wynnewood, PA.

Rev. Albert Davis, Bryn Mawr Hospital Foundation Board, Ardmore, PA.

Paul DeLomba, Mary J. Drexel Home Board, Gladwyne, PA.

Margaret H. Ewing, Main Line Health Community Services Committee; Main Line Health Board and Great Valley Health Board, West Chester, PA.

Robin Foster-Drain, M.D., To Our Children's Future with Health, Philadelphia, PA.

Barbara Hauptfuhrer, Community Services Committee of Lankenau Hospital, Stafford, PA.

John Begala, MetroHealth System, Cleveland, OH.

Marjorie Buchanan, Independence Foundation, Philadelphia, PA.

Martha Campbell, The James Irvine Foundation, San Francisco, CA.

Mike Christenson, Allina Foundation, Minneapolis, MN.

Kathryn Huschke, The Fremont Area Foundation, Fremont, MI.

Frances Jemmott, The California Wellness Foundation, Woodland Hills, CA.

Henry Jordan, M.D., Claniel Foundation, Inc., and Chester County Community Foundation, Plymouth Meeting, PA.

Linda Lloyd, Alliance Healthcare Foundation, San Diego, CA.

Thomas B. McCabe, III, Lankenau Foundation Board and Main Line Health System Board, Philadelphia, PA.

Ricardo Millet, The Kellogg Foundation, Battle Creek, MI.

Michele Murphy, McNeil Comsumer and Johnson & Johnson Foundation Board, Ft. Washington, PA.

Robin Ruben, United Way, Los Angeles, CA.

Thomas H. Sauerman, AIDS Coalition of Southern New Jersey, Philadelphia, PA.

Judy Spiegel, California Community Foundation, Los Angeles, CA.

May Anne Stetzer, Lankenau Hospital Foundation Board, Bryn Mawr, PA.

Faye Weinstein, Los Angeles Regional Family Planning Council, Los Angeles, CA.

George Weiner, The MetroHealth System, Cleveland, OH.

Nancy Whitelaw, Henry Ford Health System, Detroit, MI.

David R. Wilmerding, Jr., Lankenau Hospital Foundation Board, Rosemont, PA.

Chapter One

INTRODUCTION

In recent years, clinical decisions on patient care have come to rely more and more on the best available scientific evidence regarding the effectiveness of a given procedure or drug. How might the evidence-based approach be adapted to support decisionmaking for community-based health interventions? Would such an approach be feasible and helpful? In this report, we seek to answer these questions.

By community-based (or population-based) interventions we mean those initiated outside traditional clinical settings such as hospitals or clinics and that are primarily aimed at promoting health or preventive health practices at the community level. Most of these interventions are intended to change behavior, although some may focus on screening for undetected clinical problems. We envision such interventions as those traditionally undertaken by public health departments, "community" offices of hospitals, private health care systems including health maintenance organizations (HMOs), community-based organizations, or even churches. They might include parenting classes run by a community-based organization, radio announcements to discourage smoking, or a program at a senior center that promotes mammography screening. We recognize, however, that there is not a clean line of demarcation between clinical interventions and community interventions, and the classification of some programs as community-based may be arbitrary. For example, inoculation programs administered in health care settings would be considered clinical. However, public service announcements for a "flu" shot clinic would be community based.

Community-based interventions are funded by public health departments; federal, state, or local governments; and private foundations or other private sources of funding. We are primarily interested in private funders, such as foundations, and private health care systems. We chose not to address public agencies, such as health departments, because we hypothesized that the pressures to evaluate and fund programs would be more complex and different for public agencies than for private funding institutions.

We begin by proposing a process for deciding which community-level health programs to implement, based primarily on the strength of scientific evidence that an intervention will work and is cost-effective (see Chapter Two). Inherent in such an approach is the rigorous application of scientific principles to the ongoing evaluation of programs after they are implemented.

To help in assessing the feasibility of the approach we propose, we conducted a broad review of the literature in search of evidence on the cost and effectiveness of community health interventions (see Chapter Three). Without such evidence, of course, an evidence-based approach would not be immediately practicable.

To gain further information on the feasibility of our approach and on its utility, we conducted focus groups and telephone interviews with funders and health care organizations (Chapters Four and Five). We wanted to learn how they make decisions about community-level interventions, how much importance they accord to evidence on effectiveness and cost, and what further information they would like.

We found that the evidence currently available and the level of effort now made to generate more of it fall well short of that needed to sustain an evidence-based approach to making decisions about community health interventions. To bridge that gap, we formulated a series of recommendations for health care systems and public and private funders of health interventions (Chapter Six). These recommendations suggest steps toward applying an evidence-based approach.

Chapter Two

AN EVIDENCE-BASED APPROACH TO DECISIONMAKING FOR COMMUNITY HEALTH INTERVENTIONS

The evidence-based approach to decisionmaking was developed in the context of clinical medicine as an outgrowth of changes in medical research practices, research findings from health services research, and pressures in the health policy arena. The most important prerequisite to the development of an evidence-based approach was the acceptance of randomized clinical trials (RCTs) in clinical medical research as the "gold standard" for evaluating the effectiveness of clinical interventions. Although other forms of evidence are used to evaluate clinical interventions, it is clear that the medical research community places highest value on evidence derived from RCTs. The growth in RCTs resulted in an explosion in the volume of high-quality (if sometimes conflicting) published research about the effectiveness of clinical interventions. Furthermore, numerous studies of the use of health services documented large, unexplained variations in medical practices, suggesting a large amount of unnecessary and even harmful utilization of medical procedures and treatments. At the same time, the public sector came under increasing pressure to curb the growth of medical costs, some of which was attributed to unnecessary utilization. Critically analyzed and synthesized evidence led to the development of guidelines to help physicians make decisions for individual patients. Advocates of this evidence-based approach to medicine have emphasized its potential to reduce variation in procedure use, improve patient outcomes, and reduce costs.

The paradigm of evidence-based medicine (EBM), developed largely by clinical researchers in Canada and England, has been described as the "conscientious, explicit, and judicious use of current best evidence in making decisions about the care of individual patients" (Sackett et al., 1996). There are five elements to the paradigm (Sackett and Rosenberg, 1995):

1. Clinical and other health care decisions are based on the best patient-level, population-based, and laboratory evidence.
2. The clinical problem, rather than habits, protocols, and traditions, determines the nature and source of evidence to be sought.
3. Identifying the best evidence calls for the integration of epidemiological and biostatistical ways of thinking with those derived from pathophysiology and personal experience.
4. The conclusions of this search for and critical appraisal of evidence are worthwhile only if they are translated into actions that affect patients.
5. Providers continuously evaluate performance.

Evidence-based medicine has become a major force in U.S. health care. It is now an integral part of many stages of physicians' training. Several publications, including *Evidence-Based Medicine* and *ACP Journal Club*, are now devoted exclusively to the use of the paradigm in the critical review of medical literature. Professional organizations and the federal government have supported the development of practice guidelines based on best evidence to help physicians make clinical decisions. Yet, the EBM approach has not been without its critics. The approach has been called "elitist" (Anonymous, 1995) and "fool's gold" (Kernick, 1997), accused of implicitly denigrating the value of clinical experience and promoting "cookbook" medicine, and, perhaps most threatening, of being misused by health care managers to reduce costs. Although promoters of EBM have relied on RCTs as the "best evidence," there is debate about the true value of randomized controlled trials over other experimental designs (e.g., Herman, 1995). It is too early to assess the total effect of EBM on the health of patients and the efficient use of resources, but EBM, in some form, is likely to remain a force in clinical medicine for the foreseeable future.

Why are we interested in applying the EBM approach to the community setting? The answer is relatively straightforward and, we believe, compelling. First, with the spread of managed care, health care systems are becoming increasingly oriented toward caring for defined populations rather than individual patients. This shift in focus may force health care systems to consider implementing comprehensive health-promoting population- or community-level interventions as a natural and potentially cost-effective complement to individual health services. Many of the most costly health care problems are intimately tied to health-related behaviors, such as smoking and exercise. Community health interventions may be a cost-effective way to promote changes in many such behaviors before individuals enter the health care system with clinical disease.

Second, with the push to control costs, health care systems will face growing pressures for choosing wisely in allocating their limited resources to promote health. Most large health care systems are already involved in a range of community-based health interventions, although typically these programs are not considered an integral part of their primary mission. An evidence-based approach may help in directing increasingly scarce resources to activities that, in fact, have their desired effect and are efficient.

Third, there is evidence of a growing gap in health between those with high socioeconomic status and those with low socioeconomic status (e.g., Pappas et al., 1993). Furthermore, as health care systems, third-party insurers, and government agencies face tighter resource limitations, access to health care is likely to become more difficult for certain populations, particularly the uninsured and, among those, immigrants. Foundations and other funders may feel motivated to try closing some of these gaps and, like other health care funders, will want to make the most of what they have. They will thus also need evidence of what works best among preventive community interventions. (Foundations may also feel attracted to the evidence-based approach for no other reason than that other health care funders and policymakers are using it more, thus establishing it as the state of the art in decisionmaking.)

Although others have called for greater use of scientific evidence in making decisions about community health interventions (Muir Gray, 1997a, 1997b; Thacker et al., 1994), we noted the need for a clearer statement of principles underlying such an approach. What should be the ingredients of an evidence-based approach to making decisions about community health interventions? We propose six core underlying principles, the first five of which are adapted from the EBM approach described above.

1. Decisions about community health interventions should be drawn from the best population-based, patient-specific, and laboratory evidence.

Although we are concerned here about the role of community-based interventions exclusively, the evidence from clinical trials and laboratory work remains relevant. For example, promoting screening for hypertension is intimately tied to clinical evidence of the effectiveness of treatment for the prevention of complications. Epidemiological data can help quantify potential health benefits of interventions. Population-based data should include information on health status and health care utilization as well as social and economic conditions that are important causal forces in public health.

2. Population characteristics should determine the nature and source of evidence to be sought rather than institutional habits, protocols, traditions, or intuition.

In EBM, a clinical problem determines the search for evidence. As a unit, however, communities and populations typically do not "present" clinical problems. Indeed, the goal of most community health interventions is to prevent clinical problems. Thus, the search for evidence is inherently more difficult in the community setting, but it should be directed by the characteristics of the population. Community epidemiological studies can provide the relative importance of morbidities and risk factors in the community of interest, so that decisions involving tradeoffs across different kinds of community health problems can be tailored to a specific community.

3. Applying the best evidence calls for the integration of epidemiological and biostatistical ways of thinking with those derived from the biological, social, and behavioral sciences and from community experience, along with other community-level considerations such as equity.

Critical analysis of evidence will rarely yield a definitive answer for decisions about specific health interventions in specific communities. Each intervention and health problem is different, each community unique. Application of data to specific settings will vary. Furthermore, analyses of effectiveness and costs cannot readily incorporate important community considerations such as how the benefits of interventions are distributed within a community. Applying the evidence-based approach to community settings will require the integration of the best evidence about the effectiveness and costs of interventions with scientific knowledge of behavior and knowledge of specific communities' goals, resources, and even values. For example, the extensive experimental behavioral literature can tell us much about how and how not to change behavior.

4. The search for and critical appraisal of evidence are worthwhile only if they are translated into actions that affect communities or populations.

Obviously, if evidence does not affect decisions that in turn affect actions, the whole process is pointless.

5. Health care systems, communities, and funders should continually evaluate performance in applying these ideas.

Because each community and each setting is different, there is no guarantee that interventions proven to be effective in a research setting will work in another setting. Thus, this approach requires developing practicable methods for health care systems, communities, and funders to assess the ongoing effectiveness of interventions in their specific settings.

Beyond these five principles, application of an evidence-based approach to community health interventions presents additional challenges. Because these interventions are undertaken at a community rather than an individual level, the ability to assess and compare interventions along multiple dimensions is especially important. Physicians who apply the EBM approach may begin with the question: What is the best thing to do for this patient in this setting? But what is best for an individual patient may not be what is best from a community perspective. Communities, health care systems, and funders face limited resources and must often make choices among competing options if they are to have the maximum benefit to health in the community. Thus, an evidence-based approach at the community level must enable the assessment of resource use (costs) as well as benefits (effectiveness) across potential interventions.[1] Only by using such a broad range of evidence will it be possible to provide guidance that is as helpful to community-related decisionmaking as practice guidelines are to physicians making clinical decisions. Therefore, we add the following principle to the preceding five:

6. *The relevant scientific evidence for comparing community health interventions should encompass evidence on both the effectiveness of the interventions and their costs in a population. It should also take into account the distribution of risk factors in a community.*

In summary, we propose these six principles as the core of an evidence-based approach to decisionmaking for community health interventions.

---

[1] Whether EBM itself also includes consideration of balancing costs and benefits is the subject of debate in the literature. Maynard (1997a, 1997b) has criticized it for not doing so, but Sackett and colleagues, the leading proponents of EBM, contend that it can and does incorporate population-level perspectives such as economic analyses (Sackett et al., 1996). Clancy and Kamerow (1996) believe that EBM is defined narrowly and targeted toward clinicians, whereas cost-effectiveness analysis is targeted toward policymakers responsible for population-level choices.

Chapter Three

IS THERE ENOUGH EVIDENCE TO SUPPORT AN EVIDENCE-BASED APPROACH?

An evidence-based approach requires evidence, and the primary source of scientific evidence is the published literature. We undertook a broad review of the evaluation and effectiveness research literature to determine whether it can support evidence-based decisionmaking for community-based health interventions. Because we were interested in the "state of the art" we focused the review on evaluation of programs in the United States in the past 15 years, and we attempted to identify studies of effectiveness and studies of costs. In conducting the review, we sought to understand better how community-based programs were evaluated and what criteria of effectiveness or success were used in the published literature. Furthermore, we wanted to approximate what would happen if an informed community organization were to attempt to apply an evidence-based approach to deciding which community-based health programs to initiate.

Before summarizing the procedures we used and our findings, we address a number of limitations to our review. First, our literature review includes only evaluations that have been published. It is thus probably biased toward evaluations of high-visibility programs or those conducted by evaluators who routinely publish in the academic literature. Furthermore, we may have excluded programs that failed to achieve their initial goals if unsuccessful projects are, as many believe, less likely to be published.

Second, we did not attempt a comprehensive literature review of community-based health interventions analogous to the systematic clinical literature reviews and formal meta-analyses central to the evidence-based medicine approach (Mulrow et al., 1997; Hunt and McKibbon, 1997; Bero and Jadad, 1997; Cook et al., 1997; Sackett and Rosenberg, 1995; L'Abbe et al., 1987). Our goals were too broad to apply such an approach rigorously. Nevertheless, we have used published protocols for systematic reviews and meta-analyses as guides for our search.

Third, we excluded clinical interventions from consideration. Thus, most interventions requiring clinical staff such as immunization programs and prenatal interventions, which might be undertaken by a community group or health system, were not reviewed.

Finally, resource limitations undoubtedly resulted in our missing a number of important and relevant publications over the time period we targeted. Even narrowly defined MEDLINE literature searches focusing on clinical trials of specific interventions may miss up to half of published trials (Dickersin et al., 1994). By polling senior investigators in the field and applying other standard methods, a more intensive review might capture missed published papers, studies that were not published in venues included in computerized databases, or unpublished evaluations. Nevertheless, we believe the results of our broad review provide important insights into the obstacles that currently exist for the application of an evidence-based approach in this new arena.

METHOD

The literature review was divided into five tasks:

1. **Initial search for community-based health program articles.** We used the built-in search capabilities of two computerized commercial literature databases. We searched the HEALTH PLAN database (1980-present), which includes all health services research literature, and a majority of the relevant literature from MEDLINE. Keywords for the search were community, health intervention, evaluation, effectiveness, and cost (and combinations thereof). Articles matching those key words were downloaded into the bibliographic software package ProCite (R), which allowed us to manage and print full citations and (where available)

abstracts. The bulk of this task was conducted in December 1996. We updated it in February 1997 and added those parts of MEDLINE that are excluded from HEALTH PLAN.

2. **Keyword search of task 1 output to identify articles discussing cost, cost-effectiveness, effectiveness, or evaluation.** The task 1 search netted over 2,000 articles, so we screened on a smaller set of keywords. This cut the citation listing down to 1,067 citations.

3. **Review of citations and (where available) abstracts and rating of each article as to whether or not it should be included in an in-depth review.** For each article in the task 2 output list, we printed the full citation, which often included an abstract. All three authors reviewed the citations to determine whether or not the full paper should be obtained and a more detailed review completed. For this "gross" review, we used a series of simple inclusion and exclusion criteria (Table A.1, Appendix A). To assess the reliability of these criteria, we selected one-year of citations (1996) and compared our ratings ("yes," "no," or "maybe"). All three authors agreed on the ratings of 42 percent and two of three agreed on another 49 percent. We discussed each of the citations for which there was not complete agreement. The discussion produced consensus and on that basis we added items to the inclusion and exclusion criteria. In addition, we determined that there were certain review articles or editorials that should be obtained for background but not further reviewed for the literature search.

The output of this task was a list of 119 intervention studies and review articles (see Appendix A). Sixteen of these articles could not be located, leaving a total of 103 that were copied for in-depth review. Of these, 19 were review articles, leaving a total of 84 articles thought to be studies of community health interventions that might be useful in applying an evidence-based approach.

4. **Development of criteria for the in-depth review.** The focus of our review was on scientific evidence, specifically evidence of effectiveness of community-based health interventions. Thus, for an article to be considered as "relevant," the study had to include at least a quasi-experimental design with either a simultaneous comparison group or before-after comparisons for an intervention group. It also had to have a description of the intervention and a quantitative outcome measure. We also included general

health screening studies aimed at identifying clinical conditions among members of the community.

5. **In-depth review of articles according to criteria from Task 4.** The articles reviewed in detail were classified as relevant in applying an evidence-based approach or not. Of the 84 intervention studies identified and obtained in task 3, a total of 30 articles met our relevance criteria.

FINDINGS

We summarized the final 30 articles along several dimensions, namely, target population, setting, area of health focus, study design, and outcomes measured (see Table A.2, Appendix A). In terms of target population, about two-thirds of the interventions targeted children or adolescents with the remaining spread among the elderly, the general population, young adults, and subpopulations with specific diseases. About half of the interventions were implemented in an educational setting—a primary or secondary school or college. The remainder were either broad community interventions (e.g., public health promotion media campaigns) or were implemented at community-based organizations (e.g., Boys and Girls Clubs).

The focus of most community health interventions was on behaviors that affect health. The specific behaviors of interest varied widely across the studies, with drug and alcohol abuse being most common; others included injuries and violence, HIV prevention, cardiovascular risks, nutrition and weight loss, and exercise. For example, one strong study assessed the effect of a community-wide intervention program using a range of strategies to reduce alcohol-impaired driving, related driving risks, and traffic deaths and injuries (Hingson et al., 1996). Two studies evaluated health screening and promotion projects whose primary goal was identification of disease rather than behavioral change (Brink and Nader, 1984; Rogers et al., 1992). Although these projects were implemented in community settings, they perhaps should have been eliminated from our review because of their more clinical focus.

The most common study design was a quasi-experimental, pre-/post-intervention comparison between one or more intervention groups and a control group. However, a substantial minority of the studies involved randomization between experimental and control groups, usually at the level of the class, school, or school district or, less commonly, the community. A smaller number of studies made only a pre/post comparison for an intervention group.

A broad range of outcome measures was used to assess the effect of interventions. The most common outcomes were measures of knowledge and self-reported behavior. For example, another strong study assessed the effect of a school intervention with and without a connected media intervention designed to reduce smoking among students in grades four through six (Flynn et al., 1994). The outcome in this study was self reports of cigarettes smoked within a week of a survey. A substantial minority of studies included objective measures of health outcomes such as incidence of injuries or cholesterol and blood pressure measures. For example, an evaluation of the Stanford Adolescent Heart Health Program measured self-reported behavior such as exercise and diet as well as body mass index and resting heart rate (Killen et al., 1989). Aside from studies focusing on injuries, none measured markers of incidence of conditions such as HIV transmission rates.

Only one of the 30 articles included an analysis of costs (Rogers et al., 1992). The intervention in this study consisted of a clinical community-based program of health examinations and screenings combined with case management and education. The investigators calculated average direct monthly costs per participant over a two-year period. No other costs such as indirect costs of a participant's time were included in this analysis. Two other studies reported some measures of cost, although no detailed analyses (Hingson et al., 1996; Mayer et al., 1992). In describing the interventions evaluated, several studies reported details such as staffing requirements that could be of limited help in assessing resource requirements. In one study, a community-based weight reduction intervention was specifically described as a "low-cost" alternative to more expensive clinic-based interventions without providing any evidence of having actually assessed costs (Del Prete et al., 1993).

Typically, success was measured in terms of a statistically significant difference either between intervention and control groups or before and after the intervention. Relatively few studies discussed in detail the meaning of the magnitude of the difference in outcome measures between the intervention and the control. Only two of the papers clearly stated that the evaluation had concluded that the intervention had not had any of the desired effects (Emery and Gatz, 1990; O'Brien and Anderson, 1987). One other study concluded that the intervention had not had an effect on one of its primary outcomes (McLoughlin et al., 1982).

The studies varied considerably in the level of detail provided on the content of the intervention. Many referred to other publications for details about the intervention, but most did not themselves provide detailed descriptions.

Of the 54 articles read for the in-depth review but considered not very relevant to applying an evidence-based approach, a substantial number were found to be review articles that were not identified as such in the task 3 screening. Some of these articles might be very useful for pointing to specific examples to review in more detail or for synthesizing a large body of research, but they typically did not provide detailed information on each intervention. Several were very general and often contained only vague discussions of public policy about specific types of interventions. Several papers addressed methodologic issues in the evaluation of community health interventions.

A small number of the papers in this category were labeled as formal process or qualitative evaluations. We found these very difficult to assess. Attributions about specific results of interventions were often not backed by sufficient evidence to warrant acceptance of the conclusion. For example, one study of a community-based health promotion program stated that "churches tended to be the most effective means of reaching the target audience," yet offered no evidence to support that claim (Doyle et al., 1989). Many of these studies focused on describing what was done rather than on providing evidence of effect; some provided no evidence, quantitative or qualitative, of effect. None of the evaluations in this category involved any comparison between a control group (either pre/post or simultaneous) and the intervention participants.

DISCUSSION

The literature search for effectiveness research on community-based health interventions yielded a wide range of papers, a minority of which would be immediately useful in applying an evidence-based approach to decisionmaking for community health interventions. Only one of the papers considered relevant included an analysis of costs, and that was relatively crude. The review raised a number of important issues regarding the feasibility of applying an evidence-based approach in this setting.

Scientific Rigor of Evaluation and Effectiveness Research

Any comprehensive review of the scientific literature must ultimately make judgments about the validity of scientific findings. If, as in clinical reviews, randomized trials are accepted as the gold standard because of their ability to reduce bias, the literature in this field for the most part does not meet this standard. Perhaps this should not be surprising, as randomization for community health interventions may be more difficult than randomization of patients in a clinical setting. The exception to this generalization may be schools, and these were indeed the most common setting where randomization at the population level did occur. Attention should be given to recent calls for broader use of randomization to increase the strength of scientific evidence in community health research (Green, 1997; Fortmann et al., 1995; Green et al., 1995; Koepsell et al., 1992). At the same time, the difficulty of randomization in community interventions should also lead to more careful consideration of ways in which strong evidence regarding effect might be drawn from quasi-experimental designs. While in the clinical research setting considerable effort has been devoted to developing a consensus about a paradigm for ranking of scientific evidence (e.g., Guyatt et al., 1995), we found little evidence that such effort has occurred in the area of community health research.[1]

---

[1] Indeed, there is considerable ambiguity even about the terms we have used in our review. The investigators began the review with the assumption that evaluation research included studies of effectiveness. However, surveys suggest that evaluation research may be considered to be distinct from research to determine effectiveness (Carpinello et al., 1992).

Even more difficult than deciding what to make of quasi-experimental designs is deciding what to make of qualitative or process evaluations of community health interventions. We recognize that some effort has been devoted to the development of criteria for assessing the scientific validity of qualitative research on interventions (e.g., Muir Gray, 1997a). Process evaluations play an important role in understanding how interventions work in real communities (Goodman et al., 1993). They may also provide evidence of the effect of interventions on outcomes that are difficult to measure (Light and Pillemer, 1984), such as cultural orientation of communities toward health promotion activities. Nevertheless, we believe that these evaluations are of limited use in an evidence-based model. Without clearer guides for assessing this type of evidence, it is extremely difficult to judge the scientific validity of claims made in such analyses.

Assessing prevention effectiveness requires quantitatively analyzing the effect of interventions. As one standard evaluation text (Rossi and Freeman, 1993) states:

> [A]ssessing impact in ways that are scientifically plausible and that yield relatively precise estimates of net effects requires data that are quantifiable and systematically and uniformly collected.

Outcome Measures and Comparisons Across Potential Interventions

The most common outcome measure among the studies we considered relevant was self-reported behavior. This may not provide an accurate picture of behavior because participants may be inclined to give what they consider to be desired answers. Gold-standard measures of outcomes such as biochemical markers of smoking or even more remote outcomes such as morbidity are more expensive and may be inappropriate or impractical in a community setting (Fishbein, 1996; Mittlemark et al., 1993). Therefore, proximal measures, such as measures of behavioral change, are reasonable outcomes for most community health interventions. Nevertheless, the strength of the evidence of community health interventions will almost certainly improve with the broadened use, when feasible, of more objective and valid measures of the desired outcomes. Our review suggests the need for readily available and comprehensive guides as to the appropriateness of various outcome measures for different types of community health interventions. Such standards would facilitate assessing the evidence of effectiveness in these settings.

Even in the studies we considered relevant that used valid measures of effect, measures of similar outcomes varied with the study and typically, resource use was not reported. This impedes substantive comparisons across interventions or explicit comparisons of costs versus effectiveness or benefit. For example, if a community-based organization wanted to choose between a school-based intervention targeted at drug abuse and a community-wide intervention to target HIV prevention, the literature as it currently exists would not provide much guidance. The use of standard outcome measures and the provision of cost data would substantially improve the ability of a community-based organization to make such choices.

Access to Information on Implementation

Even if a community-based organization were to identify in the literature an intervention that it wished to implement, it might have difficulty locating details about it. Often, there appeared to be no easy way to obtain information on how to implement the programs described in the studies short of attempting to contact the authors or funding agencies directly. (It might be an interesting exercise to try to find detailed information about how to implement some of these interventions.)

The difficulty of ready access to information on implementation has been recognized as a major problem in promoting community health interventions. The Health Resources and Services Administration of the U.S. Department of Health and Human Services recently published a compendium of primary care health programs entitled *Models That Work* (Bureau of Primary Health Care, 1995). One aim of this publication (which was not identified in our literature searches) was to improve the dissemination of information about successful interventions to local organizations by providing general descriptions and addresses for program contacts. Of note, the interventions were chosen by an advisory panel of health professions and are described as "cost-effective" in the publication, but the publication unfortunately gives no rigorous evaluation of cost or effectiveness evidence. Nevertheless, publications such as this are an important step in the direction of implementing an evidence-based approach to decisions regarding community health interventions.

Chapter Four

THE VIEW FROM HEALTH CARE SYSTEMS AND FUNDERS: FOCUS GROUPS

We interviewed staff of health care systems and funders to secure additional information on the feasibility of an evidence-based approach in the community context[1] and to learn about their current use of, and need for, scientific information. We conducted our interviews both through focus groups and through one-on-one telephone conversations to exploit the advantages of each format. The give and take of focus groups permits participants to refine their positions in response to comment and may allow the development of a degree of consensus. Telephone interviews are typically less costly and more convenient for the person interviewed and permit the expression of views without regard to how other interviewees might react.

METHOD

Four focus groups were conducted—one in Los Angeles of foundation program staff, and three in the Philadelphia area of foundation program staff, foundation board members, and foundation-funded community-based program staff. The focus groups in Philadelphia were thus more heterogeneous with respect to the work roles of participants. Six to eight participants were recruited for each of the four groups, although actual attendance was between three and four par-

---

[1] Interviews were carried out while the literature review was under way, so results from the latter had little influence on interview protocols.

ticipants per group. All focus groups were held in the morning in facilities away from participant work sites.

Focus group discussions were moderated by one or another of us. Where possible, another author was present to co-moderate, observe, and take notes. Because we wanted the participants to feel comfortable and talk freely, only first names were used and confidentiality was assured. All discussions were audiotaped for transcription; the transcriptions were reviewed by project staff only.

A structured focus group protocol was developed to include the issues and questions that we wanted to raise with all groups (see Appendix B). Although differences among the groups resulted in distinctive deviations from the protocol, all the focus groups discussed these questions:

1. What drives funding priorities?
2. How are program funding decisions made?
3. How are programs evaluated by funding agencies?
4. What types of information or data would be useful to funders and grantees concerning community-based health program evaluation?

FINDINGS

A consistent observation across all focus groups was that currently very little scientific information is brought to bear in making community-based program funding decisions by foundations. Moreover, there is often little scientific information used in or generated from program evaluation. Indeed, for a variety of reasons, there are times when such information may prove to be undesirable or may even impede funding agency action. Thus, we observed that the movement to evidence-based decisionmaking found in the clinical arena has not yet reached community-based activities. This is not to say that funding decisions are made in a vacuum; indeed, foundations spent considerable time and effort in making funding decisions. The markers for program success, however, were often far from measures of cost-effectiveness or improved outcomes.

What Drives Funding Priorities

The focus groups included representatives of both private and public foundations. Thus, there were some differences in the types of grant-making that they could do as dictated by law and tax regulations. Apart from the legal differences, the foundations participating in the focus groups also had very different constituencies. Among the California foundations, the constituencies were generally state-wide, whereas among the Philadelphia foundations, the constituencies were more localized within the communities in which the foundations were located.

All foundations to an extent were receptive to national concerns and defined their priorities accordingly. For example, giving was directed to programs serving targeted groups such as the disadvantaged, women, children, and the elderly. Yet the implementation of these priorities varied. As explained by two participants, these priorities could be expansive:

> ... we are a public foundation ... we have to pretty much address state-wide issues, all levels of the population and all kinds of legitimate health as long as it is related to prevention and wellness ....

> ... our funding priorities are more goal oriented more aimed at what we are trying to achieve, a big kind of impressionistic picture, what would the community look like [if we funded this program] ....

For others, the priorities of the funding also provided opportunities for funding agencies to get noticed. As noted by two participants:

> ... quite frankly, part of our thrust is also with an eye to marketing ourselves so that potential donors will be attracted to the projects that we are funding and be supportive ....

> ... we certainly appreciate the public relations impact of our donations [funding] too, so what we try to do is get a little ... benefit from that [by] getting more press releases around the programs that we supported.

In defining priorities, foundations used their community ties. The Philadelphia-based foundations had diverse boards that included community members. Often these community members were able to bring those issues of grass-roots-level concern and need to the foundations for consideration. One foundation participated in a community needs assessment. Another relied on its sponsor's staff to identify worthy causes in the community. One provided opportunities for board trustees to identify and fund small, worthy programs, and another allowed foundation program staff to identify and fund such programs. However, as one participant indicated, trustee- or staff-initiated grants were vulnerable to "pet" project biases, and suggested, "we need better guidelines to make sure that's not happening."

The variety of mechanisms to identify funding priorities, however, did not change the general sentiment among the foundations: The goal of the foundation was to do good in the community. Often, this good was identified through intuition or gut reaction to observed conditions. As one person put it, "I feel it is our responsibility as people of means and opportunity to provide those means and opportunity to others." Another indicated, "we [the foundation] do well by doing good."

How Organizations Make Funding Decisions

Most foundations had some type of competitive proposal solicitation. Sometimes, proposals would be submitted in response to particular initiatives. In this case, proposals directed at addressing the same issue would be compared and the most deserving or meritorious would receive the funding. Other times, proposals would be submitted for funding without a major initiative. In this case, proposals addressing a variety of issues were reviewed and certain ones selected.

For proposals unrelated to particular initiatives, all foundations began review with some type of screening process. Some imposed legal criteria, such as restricting consideration to organizations with a 401c3 tax status. All imposed criteria that determined whether or not the submitted proposal related to the foundation's agenda. For example, foundations may have been more interested in funding programs that

- built community program capacity (e.g., funding to improve a management information system);
- were preventive in nature (e.g., immunization programs, education/socialization programs);
- were collaborative with other local agencies providing the same services; or
- addressed community needs, while providing public relations exposure for the foundation.

Proposals that did not meet any of these initial screening criteria were rejected.

We asked participants to what extent they relied on evidence, either found in the proposal or through other means, to determine if a proposed program would be effective and worthy of funding. The general consensus was that very few proposals were able to show that the proposed program would achieve the stated goals. (There were some notable exceptions where funding was requested to adapt an already proven intervention to a particular community.)

For the most part, the "evidence" that was brought to bear in making decisions was gathered not from the proposal but rather from the community/foundation "network." The "network" was often used to obtain information concerning the perceived management skills and fiscal stability of the prospective grantee. The use of outside experts was also used to inform the selection. As one participant explained:

> If . . . I don't have enough experience to fully understand what the project is seeking to accomplish I would send the proposal out to two, maybe three, expert reviewers . . . people who know that subject matter, the community or the approach, and if I have a bias I would send it out so that it won't just be my opinion that would be presented to the board.

Although final decisions were typically made by the board at its scheduled meetings, the board heavily depended on its program staff to review submissions and make funding recommendations; only rarely did a board disagree with a staff recommendation. Some boards developed procedures to provide the opportunity for more board involvement. These boards requested not only a synopsis of the recommended programs but also the full listing of submitted proposals. Thus, staff could be directed to reconsider a proposal if desired. Foundations that did not have a large program staff relied on funding subcommittees of the board to do the reviews and make recommendations. It appeared that these subcommittees worked similarly to program staff, but the amount of time and rigor extended in proposal evaluation may have been less.

Almost all participants acknowledged a reluctance to develop funding decisions solely on information about the effectiveness of a given approach. They believed that communities are uniquely knowledgeable about the problems they want to address, the challenges they face, and the resources they can bring to bear to "solve" the problem. Thus, employing only proven approaches to problem-solving would not permit the innovation that is often necessary to solve a given community's problem. Maintaining some flexibility in funding decisions thus could be important. As explained by one participant:

> ... although we tend to like established organizations that have track records, we set a certain amount of money that I would call venture capital, which is to new organizations that are proposing some innovative program, and they need to be supported to see if it works.

Program Evaluation

All foundation staff and grantees agreed that they required (or submitted) a discussion concerning program evaluation in their proposals. The rigor of the evaluations and the follow-up from the foundations, however, varied considerably.

Many participants offered that frequently neither the foundation staff nor the proposed program staff were capable of a formal evaluation. One participant explained that they try to keep the goals of an evaluation modest:

> [for proposal applicants, we ask] ... what difference will it make ultimately for their community or target population. We ask for written measurable objectives in the evaluation plan but I have to say, is it the most important criteria? Generally it's not, for a number of reasons. Most of the agencies we deal with are community based

organizations that may know their field very well; writing a measurable objective is not among their areas of expertise and quite frankly not among the expertise among the people in our foundation and in my experience among other people of other foundations.

This quote brings up the two broad goals of program evaluation discussed in the focus groups. The first concerned the evaluation of how successful a given program was in achieving its stated goals. The second concerned the evaluation of how much effect the foundation's funding had in the community.

To satisfy the first goal, discussants acknowledged that more could be done, but one participant offered the following observation:

. . . as we work in communities for example around issues such as doing violence prevention, we are really doing cutting edge work. I would say that often times there isn't a lot of data to support what it is we are trying to do. And then to put [the grantee] in touch with somebody who thinks they know how to prevent violence in their community is often a process that is fraught with all sorts of problems.

Programs and interventions focused on prevention offer evaluative challenges; many prevention programs do not produce short-term results. Thus, evaluation may consist of simply determining how many persons were exposed to the prevention initiative. Focus group participants agreed that wherever possible, it was also desired to get the number of persons that *could* be served, that is, the size of the community in need, so proportion of the population served could be used as a metric. While such production data may not provide a full picture of the effectiveness of a program, as one participant observed:

. . . however, I must admit, largely for our marketing purposes, we want the agencies to emphasize the numbers served because we want to announce it with our fund raising goals—what our community outreach goal will be . . . .

Beyond simple production statistics, foundations and programs try to obtain the cost per individual served. It was acknowledged that this was not a true cost-effectiveness measure, but it was the best that often could be obtained. But most foundations do not have access even to such rudimentary information. Thus, the calculus that many foundations engage in is simply, How much money do I have to spend to provide services to how many people? If the number seems reasonable, the program may be funded. If not, the program is not funded.

Collaboration with universities or other research organizations was discussed as a way to introduce more sophistication in program evaluations and perhaps get better data on program effectiveness. However, funding for such collaboration was not a high priority. One participant indicated that part of this reluctance was due to experience; past evaluations were complex and costly, and sometimes programs were unable to provide the requisite data for an evaluation. The lack of success with formal academic evaluations of community-based programs diminished the luster of such approaches as an evaluation gold standard.

For all foundations, the second goal—estimating the difference foundation dollars make in the community—is very important. Achieving this goal, however, was problematic for smaller foundations whose funding support or donations are pooled with other sources of funds, making it very difficult to identify the "bang" that resulted from their "buck." One individual indicated that as their foundation moved to be more aware of the effects of their giving, they would need to "own" programs, rather than provide some fraction of operating revenue to a program. This "ownership" would allow them to more closely monitor how their funds were being spent. On the other hand, such "ownership" would limit their ability to contribute to program types requiring large amounts of resources.

Finally, one participant observed that funding sources for many community-based programs are many and duplicative. This fractionation poses numerous problems for evaluation.

No matter what type of evaluation may be conducted, all foundations and programs face the issue of choosing a benchmark to use in their comparisons. Very few such benchmarks exist. One participant did mention that the Council of Foundations provides comparative information at their annual meeting, or at least some information that can be used in a self-assessment. However, no catalog of typical program-type-specific costs exists.

In summary, do foundations want better data? The answer is yes. However, there was considerable concern about the level of effort required to get better data. As one participant observed:

> But you don't want to put such a burden on the fundee that they are spending all their time collecting data and not delivering services.

Evaluations can cost large amounts of money, and often foundations and program staff would rather spend the money to serve people, even if no evidence can be obtained regarding the program's effect on the ultimate desired outcome. For very large initiatives, foundations may place a priority on evaluation and provide separate funding for it; smaller projects may not have such separate evaluation funding available to them.

Information Needed

Certainly some programs do generate data that provide useful information to the funder and the program, including information helpful to service improvement and funding decisions. Indeed, one organization instituted a routine service report card that was distributed quarterly to clients. Each client served by one of the organization's programs had the opportunity to provide feedback as to the quality and appropriateness of the services received. However, it appeared that most foundations did not receive such information and relied instead on community feedback to determine the effectiveness and quality of the services provided through the programs they funded.

SUMMARY

The movement to an evidence-based approach, as experienced in the clinical sector of health care, has not reached community-based programs. Indeed, funding decisions are often made without much evidence as to the effectiveness of the proposed approach. Most programs had little information as to the effectiveness of the services they provided, and often the only type of evaluative information available was production statistics and informal feedback.

Most foundation and program staff would welcome such data, if they would permit better funding decisions and program improvement. The linkage, however, was very important. Neither foundations nor program staff were interested in evaluations that did not provide such useful information. It was also clear that neither foundations nor program staff wanted to commit large sums of money to evaluation efforts. Many felt that the avenues of community feedback and production statistics provided sufficient information to make informed, albeit not perfect, decisions.

Chapter Five
THE VIEW FROM HEALTH CARE SYSTEMS AND FUNDERS: TELEPHONE INTERVIEWS

To augment the information gathered in the focus groups, we conducted a series of semi-structured telephone interviews with representatives from organizations funding community-based health interventions. The overall goal of the telephone interviews was similar to that of the focus groups: to learn how foundations and health systems make funding decisions about community-based health programs, and, in particular, whether they use scientific evidence in this process.

The nature of these interviews (one on one), however, allowed us to broaden the geographic scope of the organizations involved and to explore in more depth the issues raised in the focus groups. We were also interested in obtaining input from some foundations larger than most of those represented in the focus groups and thus with more funds to allocate and a broader scope of contribution. In addition to foundation representatives, we interviewed personnel from large health systems that conduct community-based health interventions and must decide how to allocate funds across a variety of projects.

METHOD

We conducted nine telephone interviews; six of these were with foundation representatives and three were with health system representatives. The organizations were in various geographic locations throughout the Midwest, the Northeast, and Southwest United

States. The main eligibility criteria for selecting individuals to interview were that

- the individual worked for an organization allocating a significant portion of its funds to community-based health interventions; and
- the representative interviewed had decisionmaking responsibility over funding decisions.

All nine participants were at similar levels within their respective organizations: the senior program officer or vice president level for the foundation representatives and the associate director or director level for the health system representatives.

Before beginning the interview, we explained the goal of our project and provided definitions for "evidence-based" and "community-based":

> By an evidence-based approach, we mean a process by which decisions are made at least partly on the strength of scientific evidence that a community-based intervention will work. We also mean the rigorous application of scientific principles to assess a program after implementation to determine whether it worked. By community-based, we mean those programs that might be conducted with local organizations at the community level that promote health or preventive health practices.

The telephone interviews were audiotaped (with the permission of the participants) and lasted approximately 45–60 minutes each. Written summaries of individual responses were prepared to identify key themes. The key themes centered on questions similar to those explored in the focus groups (see Appendix C for details):

1. What are the types of programs funded, the communities served, and the specific health issues addressed?
2. What are the processes for making decisions about funding (or doing) the programs and what factors drive these processes? To what extent is evidence used?
3. How are programs evaluated?

4. What information would be helpful to funders and health system decisionmakers concerning community-based health program evaluation?

FINDINGS

The amount of money dispersed by the foundations to community-based health programs ranged from approximately $2 million to $5 million per year. Several of the foundations had experienced significant increases in their grant-making machines, either through endowments or substantial increases in assets such as stock. Given this increase, they expressed a great deal of interest in finding "good ways to spend the money."

Types of Programs Funded

Most of the foundation representatives and all of the health system representatives focused their programs on a specific county or metropolitan area. The others had state-wide constituencies. Almost all of the organizations articulated some priority program areas, such as substance abuse, communicable diseases, violence, mental health, rural health, teen pregnancy, HIV/AIDS, diabetes, asthma, environmental health, and access to health care. Some also expressed priority for certain populations, such as the medically indigent, the underserved, the "disadvantaged," women, children, teens, and the elderly. But only a few talked about specific "strategic" priorities, i.e., longer-term goals, such as integrating health and community systems, addressing the ethics of health care delivery and finance, building models of primary prevention, and promoting healthy communities.

The majority of the foundations fund between 25 and 50 community-based health programs each. One foundation and one health system each fund around 200 programs, but some of the grants are very small. There does not seem to be a "typical" community-based health program for most of these organizations; grant sizes range from $500 to millions of dollars.

How Organizations Make Funding Decisions

There was a certain amount of consistency among the organizations in their procedures for making decisions about funding. Generally, a handful of full- and part-time staff review proposals and make recommendations to a board for final approval. Proposals are often submitted in competition with others, although it is not uncommon for foundations to seek out certain organizations or individuals to carry out a program that they feel is important. As one foundation representative explained:

> I think competitive processes are not always appropriate. There are times when you need to attract a leader, a star to a particular field of endeavor. Stars don't need to get in line in competitive processes; their time is very well cared for for years to come, so you need to actually get in line and compete for their time . . . . RFP [Requests for Proposals] and competitive processes won't necessarily attract brave people, and brave people are what you need very often to get the work done.

Other foundation representatives expressed similar sentiments. Several indicated that they actively use their contacts in the foundation world and in the community to seek out such "brave people" and organizations, to get to know the "players."

The way that foundations review proposals varies depending on the in-house expertise available and their knowledge of the applicant organization.[1] Some of the different assessment strategies include sending the proposals out for external review, conducting site visits, reviewing the organizations' financial statements and audits, and asking other funders about their knowledge and experiences with the soliciting organizations. One foundation representative explained that they have the responsibility to assess whether something is really a priority:

---

[1] Large health systems, meanwhile, find themselves increasingly playing a dual role: They receive outside funding for a particular initiative and then disperse the funds to various community-based entities for program delivery. According to one representative, this means that they take the lead and make commitments to external funding agencies but are not necessarily "the owners of the thing on the delivery side; it can be a shared process."

> Everybody has pet projects and we certainly bring our own pet projects and expertise to that table. So, when people come and say, "This is a priority," we say, "Well, is it really a priority?" It's our responsibility to go out and see, is it or isn't it? We have a very good relationship with our Department of Health Services. We know whom to call, and we call up and say, "Can you give us the stats on this?" or, "What do you think about this?" "Is it a big problem, or is it as big as they say?"

Evidence-based approaches such as cost-effectiveness analysis are not commonly used in making decisions about community-based programs, although there seemed to be great interest in getting such information. A few of those interviewed did say that they relied on cost-effectiveness, which they most often defined as cost per client served (as outlined in program proposals or financial reports). Even so, at least one of these admitted that the cost per client is not the bottom line and that for some programs the decisionmaking and evaluation tend to "respond on an emotional level" (i.e., how much "good" the program is achieving on a qualitative level). Another foundation representative acknowledged that "the managed care perspective" is causing them to pay more attention to cost-effectiveness. Foundation personnel also recognized the need for evidence if they hoped to ultimately affect policy. As one representative explained:

> If you have a particular initiative or a major, multi-site effort that wants to impact policy ... of course you want credible data. To get credible data, you have to have institutions who are participating as grantees who can deliver with organizational maturity and capacity .... Some of the pre-funding assessments will include some assessment of that organization's history on effectiveness. So effectiveness becomes a criterion that gets factored into funding decisions before and certainly a criterion that the board is interested in looking at as a result of their program experience with us.

For both foundations and health systems, funding priorities are affected by strategic planning. Those interviewed were generally committed to strategic planning, though foundations' experience with it varies. Several report relying on their board, which "represents the community," to make the decisions and "set the course." Several organizations cited examples of how they use data in planning, such as developing a profile of health problems in the county to compare them to state and national profiles to see where health problems are not being addressed. Indeed, current trends—local and national—are playing an increasing role in determining priorities. For example, managed care and health finance policy reforms were mentioned by all organizations as important factors affecting their funding priorities. It also seemed important to some that they identify needs that are not being met by other foundations and programs.

Program Evaluation

Typically, outcome-oriented statements are included in the program proposals that are then used as the basis for evaluation. And, as with program funding, foundation officials saw the need for generating evidence if they wanted to have a policy effect:

> As we, in this and in other foundations, increasingly talk about wanting to affect policy and wanting to be "players" in the policy world, there's no way you can get there unless you are able to generate data that is relevant and sufficiently rigorous to merit consideration in the policy arena. Who wants to make policy decisions on data that is shaky?

Still, many of the evaluations ultimately examine process, since many of the outcomes are long-term goals and may not be measurable during the funding period. As one foundation representative explained:

> We are very much looking at health promotion and disease prevention activities for which real health status indicators may not emerge for five to 10 years. And so, as a result, we help people try to shape their proposals in the form of programmatic impact statements, but we build in mechanisms for measurement that will set baselines and enable them to gather data that will focus on health status in three years, five years, or 10 years, so that the effectiveness of their work can be monitored. It's the classic dilemma, if you provide a two-year grant, the chances of seeing a reduction in infant mortality are slim to none in that time frame. What we do is encourage organizations to describe in their proposal and document the credibility of their intervention and its potential impact on

health status. Then we ask them to make sure that they have a monitoring system in place.

Other constraints on evaluation are the resources required to conduct outcome-oriented evaluations. There is a direct tradeoff between these kinds of evaluations and providing maximum funds for service delivery. Foundation and health system representatives with more of a research orientation try to incorporate academic rigor into their evaluations. However, they sense the need for "appropriate evaluations," i.e., evaluations that are relevant for the particular program given the organization's resources, the size of the grant, and the strategy of the program.

All the organizations we interviewed generally require some kind of written report from their programs, either through standard evaluation forms or ones that the grantees create themselves. Financial reports are standard. Production statistics (number of clients served, etc.) are also common. Site visits are used frequently to evaluate programs. At a minimum, organizations are expected to show whether they achieved their stated objectives, although foundations generally understand that this criterion does not guarantee program effectiveness. Very few of the organizations felt that they possessed the resources and capacity to "go to the next level" to assess effectiveness. One foundation, however, said that it includes a major evaluation component (approximately 20 percent of the total grant) as part of every initiative.

Several organizations prided themselves on being risk-takers, i.e., they expect that a certain number of the programs will not be successful. As one foundation representative explained:

> We call ourselves the "50 Percent Club." About 50 percent of our stuff should work, and about 50 percent of it shouldn't. If 90 percent of our stuff works, then we're not taking enough risks. If 10 percent of our stuff works, then we're taking too much risk.... So, we aim for about the 50 percent level, and then we teach ourselves to expect failure and report failure truthfully. That's a tough deal.

All organizations said that they really want to know what happened with the programs, that there is "no need for gloss," but they recognize that the grant-making system provides incentives for reporting only successes. This places pressure on the programs funded as well as the foundation program officers who oversee these projects:

> Part of the challenge has been to allay the anxiety of the program officers that the Board would only want to learn about successful programs. Naturally, program officers want to look as good as possible to their Board of Trustees. We can pay anyone to manage a failed program, but we only pay the best to manage successful programs. So there is an inordinate amount of pressure on program officers and it chills the notion that you can learn anything from failure.

Overall, the amount of evaluation required of community-based organizations is quite variable and seems to depend on the particular orientation of program staff and others involved in decisionmaking. As one foundation representative observed:

> When I talk to other foundations, I am shocked at how little evaluation is expected from [the programs they fund]. I feel that we should expect more. When I listen to some of the other foundations, ours sound like university-level stuff. I think that it is the foundations—they don't have the in-house expertise, and I think that's a problem. Because the benefit of having it, or bringing it in, is that you can tell your board where you're being successful and where you're not. And you provide a benefit to your grantee because they need to get more funding. And the only way they're going to get additional funding is if they can show that that program was successful and effective. So, on the one hand, not expecting your grantees to do a decent job in evaluating their program does not give them any advantage in the long-run. It may be easier during the year of the program, but you're not doing them any favors. The benefit in the long run is better understanding, and they'll enjoy evaluations. People are scared of that word. Foundations don't do enough in that area, and I think that's something that we need to improve.

Information Needed

There was consensus that more information is needed and that, given the managed care environment, an evidence-based approach would make sense. However, it was clear that foundations do not fund the kinds of projects that may be necessary to produce such information. One representative, however, suggested a unique role for foundations in this regard:

> It is our perspective that evidence-based initiatives are really important, but that one of the roles that foundations can play is setting up early initiatives that push the envelope a little bit and end up initiating efforts that will in fact generate the evidence that will enable them to become institutionalized in whatever way makes sense.

MEDLINE and Internet searches are often used by foundation and health system staff to gather information, but, as discussed in Chapter Three, it is difficult to make a case for the cost-effectiveness of any approach through the published literature. Increasingly, organizations that fund community-based health interventions seem to be partnering with academic and research institutions to collect such information. For example, several foundations said that they assign academic researchers to particular projects with the idea that the researcher will help the community-based organization develop appropriate evaluations. The funding for the researcher is usually provided by foundations.

When asked about what information they would like to have to evaluate program effectiveness, some of the more common responses given by the interviewees included the following:

- total program costs;
- service utilization;
- client or patient perspective (satisfaction, etc.); and
- substantive health status indicators and measures of desired intervention outcomes.

Overall, those interviewed acknowledged the lack of useful information available to them for evaluating program effectiveness. And although all conceded that their decisionmaking would improve with additional information,[2] they expressed some ambivalence about

___
[2] Provided it is of the right kind. Representatives of health care systems told us they are collecting so much information now that a principal need is help in figuring out what to make of it.

how realistic an evidence-based approach is for most community-based interventions. They also stressed the importance of judgment and "street sense" in making sound decisions about community health interventions. Nevertheless, the imperative for an evidence-based approach was recognized at some level by all those interviewed. As one representative explained:

> There is an absence of "real life research." It involves asking the questions in a plain and simple manner and comparing the cost-effectiveness of community investments from many different disciplines. For example, you can raise immunization rates by advertising on TV, by distributing free vaccines, by appearing at grocery stores, by asking physicians to be more orderly in their protocol. Which one should you invest in? The answer to that is: Real life research doesn't crawl into a department or division in an academic health center. It asks the question plainly and simply: "If you have a certain amount of money, how is it best invested?"

SUMMARY

Funders and health system managers involved in community-based health interventions have established procedures for screening applicants and evaluating programs that involve a variety of inputs: expert review, building the organizational capacity to self-evaluate, and fostering collaborations between community-based programs and academic institutions. They are responsive to community input through board representation and "being out there" in the community (networking, getting to know the "players," etc.).

Overall, there was great interest in using evidence to guide funding decisions and the evaluation of community-based health interventions. But for foundation and health system personnel the prevailing understanding of evidence-based approaches is variable. For example, several interviewees used the term "cost-effectiveness approaches" to refer to cost per client served. In the absence of other information, those we interviewed relied on production statistics and financial data that are generally available. Almost all, however, expressed interest in information that would allow them to measure effectiveness at a more sophisticated level.

The challenges of developing an evidence-based approach for community health interventions are several. First, the outcomes of such programs involve multiple levels (individual and community) and may not always be easily isolated for measurement. Second, long-term outcomes to inform present decisionmaking may not be available. Finally, community programs find themselves in a precarious position: Their continued funding usually depends on program success. They may not find an evidence-based approach appealing if it threatens their existence.

Chapter Six

TOWARD AN EVIDENCE-BASED APPROACH TO COMMUNITY HEALTH INTERVENTIONS

A consistent message we received from our focus groups and telephone interviews was this: Private funders, community-based organizations, and health care systems all generally believe that they should be doing a better job in critically assessing interventions they fund and implement. They also generally welcome the use of a more scientific approach to decisionmaking. We believe that an evidence-based approach analogous to EBM can work as an organizing framework for promoting the use of scientific evidence in making decisions about community health interventions. But we also know that there are many obstacles to the immediate application of such an approach in this setting.

We found the literature seriously wanting in its relevance to a rigorous evidence-based approach. Our review of the literature suggests, first, that relatively few rigorous evaluations of community health interventions are published in the indexed journals. Second, we confirmed that almost no cost analyses of community health interventions are published. What Maynard (1997b) noted about the evidence on assessment of clinical interventions appears to be equally true for community health interventions:

> . . . all too little cost data have been collected and in many cases their accuracy is dubious. Economic evaluation is in a pubescent state, rather like clinical trial practice several decades ago.

If an evidence-based approach to decisionmaking for community health interventions cannot be immediately implemented, what might be done to facilitate its future realization? In answering this question, it is important to reconsider the conditions that contributed to the growth of the evidence-based approach in clinical settings:

- the wide acceptance in the scientific community of the randomized clinical trial as the gold standard of evidence of clinical efficacy;
- a large body of motivating data about the use of health care services, especially on small-area variations in use that did not appear to be explained by variations in need;
- growing economic pressure to control health care costs: Averting unnecessary use of services or the use of unproved services held out the potential for reducing costs, though the evidence of such an effect is still limited;
- capitated reimbursement financing mechanisms for exerting economic pressures for increased efficiency;
- the changing structure of the delivery system for clinical care, especially the growth of HMOs, which provided an organizational framework for imposing the new EBM approach on physicians;
- the growing threat of liability, which may also have encouraged acceptance of EBM because of the potential for providing a clearer standard of care; and
- strong support for change by leading health care organizations such as the American Medical Association and the American College of Physicians and journals such as *JAMA*, *Annals of Internal Medicine*, and the *British Medical Journal*.

We do not see the same factors promoting the evolution of an evidence-based approach in the community context:

- There is no widely accepted gold standard for scientific evidence of the effectiveness and costs of community-level interventions. A framework for helping decisionmakers in community settings assess evidence would be a necessary and important first step toward wider use of evidence in decisionmaking. Such a framework would promote consistency in the assessment of evidence and guidelines for organizations with limited in house scientific expertise.

- In contrast to the clinical setting, where there is a large body of evidence on rates of service and procedure use and variations in practice, there are few data on the universe of community-based health interventions, for example, rates, funding, variation across communities, costs, types, and effects. Thus, there is little empirical motivation to suggest inefficient use of resources.

- There is no centralized system of funding of community health interventions that provides a financial mechanism for increasing incentives for doing a better job. The decisionmakers for community-level interventions are diffuse—they include public health departments, insurers and HMOs, foundations, community-based organizations, and hospitals. Each of these brings a different perspective to the choices to be made.

- Though at a system level the pressure to prevent costly illness may be growing, the incentives to do so remain ambiguous at the population level for health care systems such as HMOs. For example, the chronic illnesses that an HMO wishes to prevent may not appear for many years after an intervention. Thus, patients may be cared for by another HMO when the benefit of prevented illness occurs. Although most health care plans may be genuinely motivated to promote health in their populations even without evidence of direct economic benefits, clearer short-term economic evidence and incentives would strengthen this desire.

- Although there is a widespread belief that community-level health interventions will lower costs for health care systems, there is, in fact, little evidence supporting that conclusion.

- There is often no clear health "problem" that serves as a starting point for triggering a response analogous to a patient who presents to a doctor with a specific clinical problem. The motivation is often not to solve a specific problem but simply to do good, to promote the general health of a population (and, only recently, to do so efficiently).

- Thus far, no leaders have taken up the call to promote an evidence-based approach in decisionmaking for community-level health interventions.

Some of these factors will not change in the foreseeable future. For example, the benefits of community health interventions will probably remain distant and there will thus be few assurances that they will accrue to the health care systems that invest in those programs. As a result, there will almost certainly continue to be only loose economic incentives for such "investors."

However, steps can be taken to move toward an evidence-based approach. In looking toward these steps, we focus on the role of health care systems that are engaged in community health interventions and that would like to make better choices and foundations and other private funders of many local community health interventions. Many of the suggestions we make that are geared toward private funders apply equally to public health departments at the state or local level and the federal government, but a more detailed discussion of their roles is beyond the scope of this report.

HEALTH CARE SYSTEMS

1. Allocate a portion of the budget for community-based interventions to those for which there is quantitative evidence of effectiveness and, when possible, efficiency. For example, we located a substantial body of literature about the effectiveness of various school-based health promotion interventions from which reasonable choices could be made. Obviously, our literature review suggests that there is only a limited range of interventions for which there is good evidence of effectiveness, and an even more limited range for cost-effectiveness. Nevertheless, this step might send an important message of the need for better evidence.

2. Develop broad-based community-wide coalitions including health care systems, community-based organizations, and public health departments to coordinate community-wide strategies for implementation and evaluation of health interventions. This might make evidence-based approaches more feasible because evaluation costs could be shared across a number of entities.

3. Partner with academic, research, and other health care organizations to promote rigorous analyses and evaluations of interventions. Such a partnership might take the form of a long-term commitment between a health care system or a coalition of sys-

tems and a university. The commitment would involve support for researchers, integration of researchers into making decisions about community-level health interventions, and joint applications for funding of interventions and evaluations.

4. Begin to collect data on costs of all interventions.

5. Incorporate into requests for external funds as much as feasible the best evidence that the proposed interventions will work.

PRIVATE FUNDERS

1. Support the formation of a consortium to establish standards and guidelines for the assessment of evidence regarding effectiveness and costs of community-based health interventions. The resultant consensus guidelines would be used by organizations that are attempting to employ an evidence-based approach to choosing interventions and by organizations that are initiating interventions and wish to rigorously assess their effect. Such guidelines should address appropriate measures of outcomes for various types of interventions and components of a "minimum data set," which all community health interventions should collect. Development of such consensus-based guidelines could reduce the costs to individual funders who wish to use an evidence-based approach in their funding activities.

2. Promote more rigorous evaluations of interventions by funding evaluations, especially the collection of meaningful cost data.

3. Promote the collection of data to describe the full range of community health interventions, including the types of evaluations performed, their costs, how interventions were chosen, funding patterns, and outcomes. Even detailed descriptions of the universe of health interventions undertaken in several selected communities would be informative.

4. To make data more accessible to health care systems and community-based organizations, promote the establishment of centralized sources of information on community-based interventions and evidence of effectiveness and costs.

5. Promote the formation of regional coalitions that can provide technical assistance (including help in evaluation) to community-based organizations and health care systems wanting to apply an evidence-based approach.
6. Fund research to assess the economic effect of community-based interventions on health care organizations such as HMOs.
7. Provide greater incentives for organizations to be open in disseminating evidence about interventions that do not achieve their goals. One mechanism might be the increased use of multiyear, multiproject funding for which renewal is based on quality of evaluation as well as effectiveness.
8. Provide leadership for encouraging the use of an evidence-based approach for community intervention decisionmaking. Such leadership might entail funding workshops and conferences and writing editorials that promote open discussion of the potential for such an approach to improve efficient and effective use of funds intended to promote healthy communities.

Appendix A
LITERATURE IDENTIFIED

Following are the 119 articles identified as potentially relevant in task 3 of the literature review (see Chapter Three). They include some review articles identified for background information only. Research articles that could be located were subjected to in-depth review to determine whether they provided useful cost and effectiveness evidence. Our judgment in that regard is summarized in the status indicator for each citation. The indicator shows whether the article turned out to be an evaluation or something else (e.g., needs assessment or case study), and, if an evaluation, whether it is relevant to an evidence-based approach.

1. Aiken LS, West SG, Woodward CK, Reno RR, Reynolds KD. Increasing screening mammography in asymptomatic women: evaluation of a second-generation, theory-based program. *Health Psychol.* 1994 Nov.

STATUS: NOT LOCATED[1]

2. Alfano AM, Nerviano VJ. Considerations for survival in program evaluation projects. *Int J Addict.* 1988 Jan; 23(1): 109–113.

STATUS: REVIEW/POLICY/OPINION

---

[1] These articles were not located and could not be reviewed.

3. Altman DG, Endres J, Linzer J, Lorig K, Howard-Pitney B, Rogers T. Obstacles to and future goals of ten comprehensive community health promotion projects. *J Community Health*. 1991 Dec; 16(6): 299–314.

STATUS: REQUESTED REVIEW

4. Anglin TM. Position paper on school-based health clinics. The Society for Adolescent Medicine. *J Adolesc Health Care*. 1988 Nov; 9(6): 526–530.

STATUS: REVIEW/POLICY/OPINION

5. Anspaugh DJ, Hunter S, Mosley J. The economic impact of corporate wellness programs: past and future considerations. *AAOHN J*. 1995 Apr; 43(4): 203–210.

STATUS: REQUESTED REVIEW

6. Balestreire JJ, Burdick WP, Caplan D, Carroll T, Davidson SJ, Geller A, Gerrity P, Gordon P, Morahan PS, Rawson I, Smithyman K, Varga JL. The Pennsylvania Local Interdisciplinary Team: journey into collaborative learning and community health improvement. *Jt Comm J Qual Improv*. 1996 Mar; 22(3): 171–177.

STATUS: CASE STUDY

7. Bergofsky L, Barron E, Goodwin, RE. Putting the poor first. A system's assessment project identifies community needs. *Health Prog*. 1991 Dec; 64–67, 76.

STATUS: NEEDS ASSESSMENT

8. Best JA. Intervention perspectives on school health promotion research. *Health Educ Q*. 1989 Summer; 16(2): 299–306.

STATUS: REVIEW/POLICY/OPINION

9. Braun SH, Irving D. A natural history of behavioral health program evaluation in Arizona. *Community Ment Health J.* 1984 Spring; 20(1): 56–71.

STATUS: REVIEW/POLICY/OPINION

10. Brink SG, Nader PR. Comprehensive health screening in elementary schools: an outcome evaluation. *J Sch Health.* 1984 Feb; 54(2): 75–78.

STATUS: EVALUATION—NOT RELEVANT

11. Brunk SE, Goeppinger J. Process evaluation. Assessing reinvention of community-based interventions. *Eval Health Prof.* 1990 Jun; 13(2): 186–203.

STATUS: REVIEW/POLICY/OPINION

12. Bush PJ, Zuckerman AE, Taggart VS, Theiss PK, Peleg EO, Smith SA. Cardiovascular risk factor prevention in black school children: the "Know Your Body" evaluation project. *Health Educ Q.* 1989 Summer; 16(2): 215–227.

STATUS: CASE STUDY

13. Cadman D, Chambers L, Feldman W, Sackett D. Assessing the effectiveness of community screening programs. *JAMA.* 1984 Mar 23/30 1984; 251(2): 1580–1585.

STATUS: REQUESTED REVIEW

14. Campanelli PC, Dielman TE, Shope JT, Butchart AT, Renner DS. Pretest and treatment effects in an elementary school-based alcohol misuse prevention program. *Health Educ Q.* 1989 Spring; 16(1): 113–130.

STATUS: EVALUATION—RELEVANT

15. Carpinello SE, Newman DL, Jatulis LL. Health decision makers' perceptions of program evaluation. Relationship to purpose and information needs. *Eval Health Prof.* 1992 Dec; 15(4): 405–419.

STATUS: REQUESTED REVIEW—METHODS

16. Carroccio J, Wilson L, Pryor J, Marks LN, Nippes JK. A senior volunteer/home care agency national collaboration: assessment of the partnership. *J Volunt Adm.* 1996 Summer.

STATUS: NOT LOCATED

17. Centers for Disease Control. Community-level prevention of human immunodeficiency virus infection among high-risk populations: the AIDS Community Demonstration Projects. *MMWR Morb Mortal Wkly Rep.* 1996 May 10; 45(RR6): 1–24.

STATUS: EVALUATION—RELEVANT

18. Centers for Disease Control and Prevention. Guidelines for school health programs to promote lifelong healthy eating. *MMWR Morb Mortal Wkly Rep.* 1996 Jun 14; 45(RR6): 1–41.

STATUS: REQUESTED REVIEW

19. Centers for Disease Control. School health assessment, planning, and evaluation project—New York City. *MMWR Morb Mortal Wkly Rep.* 1984 Aug 31;.33(34): 489–491.

STATUS: NEEDS ASSESSMENT

20. Cheadle A, Wagner E, Koepsell T, Kristal A, Patrick D. Environmental indicators: a tool for evaluating community-based health-promotion programs. *Am J Prev Med.* 1992 Nov–1992 Dec 31; 8(6): 345–350.

STATUS: METHODS—NOT RELEVANT

21. Cheadle A, Psaty BM, Diehr P, Koepsell T, Wagner E, Curry S, Kristal A. Evaluating community-based nutrition programs: comparing grocery store and individual-level survey measures of program impact. *Prev Med.* 1995 Jan; 24: 71–79.

STATUS: REQUESTED REVIEW—METHODS

22. Cohen RY, Felix MR, Brownell KD. The role of parents and older peers in school-based cardiovascular prevention programs: implications for program development. *Health Educ Q.* 1989 Summer; 16(2): 245–253.

STATUS: EVALUATION—RELEVANT

23. Combs-Orme T, Reis J, Ward LD. Effectiveness of home visits by public health nurses in maternal and child health: an empirical review. *Public Health Rep.* 1985 Sep/Oct 31; 100(5):490–499.

STATUS: REQUESTED REVIEW

24. Cooper JK. Accountability for clinical preventive services. *Mil Med.* 1995 Jun; 160(6): 297–299.

STATUS: REVIEW/POLICY/OPINION

25. D'Onofrio CN. Making the case for cancer prevention in the schools. *J Sch Health.* 1989 May; 59(5): 225–231.

STATUS: REVIEW/POLICY/OPINION

26. Del Prete L, English C, Caldwell M, Banspach SW, Lefebvre C. Three-year follow-up of Pawtucket Heart Health's community-based weight loss programs. *Am J Health Promot.* 1993 Jan/Feb; 7(3): 182–187.

STATUS: EVALUATION—NOT RELEVANT

27. Dielman TE, Shope JT, Leech SL, Butchart AT. Differential effectiveness of an elementary school-based alcohol misuse prevention program. *J Sch Health.* 1989 Aug; 59(6): 255–263.

STATUS: EVALUATION—RELEVANT

28. Dignan MB, Beal PE, Michielutte R, Sharp PC, Daniels LA, Young LD. Development of a direct education workshop for cervical cancer prevention in high risk women: the Forsyth County project. *J Cancer Educ.* 1990; 5(4): 217–223.

STATUS: EVALUATIONS—NOT RELEVANT

29. Dommeyer CJ, Marquard JL, Gibson JE, Taylor RL. The effectiveness of an AIDS education campaign on a college campus. *J Am Coll Health.* 1989 Nov; 38: 131–135.

STATUS: EVALUATION—RELEVANT

30. Doyle E, Smith CA, Hosokawa MC. A process evaluation of a community-based health promotion program for a minority target population. *Health Educ.* 1989 Dec; 20(5): 61–64.

STATUS: EVALUATION—NOT RELEVANT

31. Dunkle M. Asking the right questions about school health programs [comment]. *J Sch Health.* 1990 Apr; 60(4): 147–148.

STATUS: REVIEW/POLICY/OPINION

32. Dunnette DA. Assessing risks and preventing disease from environmental chemicals. *J Community Health.* 1989 Fall; 14(3): 169–186.

STATUS: REVIEW/POLICY/OPINION

33. Eisen M, Zellman GL, McAlister AL. Evaluating the impact of a theory-based sexuality and contraceptive education program. *Fam Plann Perspect.* 1990 Nov/Dec; 22(6): 261–271.

STATUS: EVALUATION—RELEVANT

34. Elder JP, Edwards CC, Conway TL, Kenney E, Johnson CA, Bennett ED. Independent evaluation of the California Tobacco Education Program. *Public Health Rep.* 1996 Jul/Aug; 111: 353–358.

STATUS: EVALUATION—NOT RELEVANT

35. Emery CF, Gatz M. Psychological and cognitive effects of an exercise program for community-residing older adults. *Gerontologist.* 1990 Apr; 30(2): 184–188.

STATUS: EVALUATION—RELEVANT

36. Evans RI, Raines BE, Owen AE. Formative evaluation in school-based health promotion investigations. *Prev Med.* 1989 Mar; 18: 229–234.

STATUS: METHODS

37. Finnegan JR Jr, Murray DM, Kurth C, McCarthy P. Measuring and tracking education program implementation: the Minnesota Heart Health Program experience. *Health Educ Q.* 1989 Spring; 16(1): 77–90.

STATUS: REQUESTED REVIEW

38. Finney JW. Enhancing substance abuse treatment evaluations: examining mediators and moderators of treatment effects. *J Subst Abuse.* 1995.

STATUS: NOT LOCATED

39. Fishbein M. Great expectations, or do we ask too much from community-level interventions? [editorial; comment]. *Am J Public Health.* 1996 Aug; 86(8): 1075–1076.

STATUS: REVIEW/POLICY/OPINION

40. Flynn BS, Worden JK, Secker-Walker RH, Pirie PL, Badger GJ, Carpenter JH, Geller BM. Mass media and school interventions for cigarette smoking prevention: effects 2 years after completion. *Am J Public Health.* 1994 Jul; 84(7): 1148–1150.

STATUS: EVALUATION—RELEVANT

41. Fors SW, Owen S, Hall WD, McLaughlin J, Levinson R. Evaluation of a diffusion strategy for school-based hypertension education. *Health Educ Q.* 1989 Summer; 16(2): 255–261.

STATUS: EVALUATION—RELEVANT

42. Fortmann SP, Flora JA, Winkleby MA, Schooler C, Taylor CB, Farquhar JW. Community intervention trials: reflections on the Stanford Five-City Project Experience. *Am J Epidemiol.* 1995 Sep 15; 142(6): 576–586.

STATUS: REVIEW/POLICY/OPINION

43. Friedman RH, Kazis LE, Jette A, Smith MB, Stollerman J, Torgerson J, Carey K. A telecommunications system for monitoring and counseling patients with hypertension. Impact on medication adherence and blood pressure control. *Am J Hypertens.* 1996 Apr.

STATUS: NOT LOCATED

44. Gainer PS, Champion HR. Unconvincing evidence for condemning school-based conflict resolution programs [comment]. *Health Aff (Millwood).* 1994 Fall; 165–167.

STATUS: REVIEW/POLICY/OPINION

45. Gans KM, Levin S, Lasater TM, Sennett LL, Maroni A, Ronan A, Carleton RA. Heart healthy cook-offs in home economics classes: an evaluation with junior high school students. *J Sch Health.* 1990 Mar; 60(3): 99–102.

STATUS: EVALUATION—RELEVANT

46. Glynn TJ. Essential elements of school-based smoking prevention programs. *J Sch Health.* 1989 May; 59(5): 181–188.

STATUS: REVIEW/OPINION/POLICY

47. Goeppinger J, Macnee C, Anderson MK, Boutaugh M, Stewart K. From research to practice: the effects of the jointly sponsored dissemination of an arthritis self-care nursing intervention. *Appl Nurs Res.* 1995 Aug; 8(3): 106–113.

STATUS: EVALUATION—RELEVANT

48. Goldman HH, Morrissey JP, Ridgely MS. Evaluating the Robert Wood Johnson Foundation program on chronic mental illness. *Milbank Q.* 1994; 72(1): 37–47.

STATUS: REVIEW/POLICY/OPINION (?CLINICAL)

49. Goodman RM, Steckler A, Hoover S, Schwartz R. A critique of contemporary community health promotion approaches: based on a qualitative review of six programs in Maine. *Am J Health Promot.* 1993 Jan/Feb; 7(3): 208–220.

STATUS: EVALUATION—RELEVANT

50. Gordis L. Evaluating the evidence for the effectiveness of prevention. *J Gen Intern Med.* 1990 Sep/Oct (Supplement); 5: S14–S16.

STATUS: REQUESTED REVIEW

51. Gregor S, Galazka, SS. The use of key informant networks in assessment of community health. *Fam Med.* 1990 Mar/Apr; 22(2): 118–121.

STATUS: METHODS

52. Guyer B, Gallagher SS, Chang BH, Azzara CV, Cupples LA, Colton T. Prevention of childhood injuries: evaluation of the Statewide Childhood Injury Prevention Program (SCIPP). *Am J Public Health.* 1989 Nov; 79(11): 1521–1527.

STATUS: EVALUATION—RELEVANT

53. Hausman AJ, Spivak H, Prothrow-Stith D, Roeber J. Patterns of teen exposure to a community-based violence prevention project. *J Adolesc Health.* 1992 Dec; 13(8): 668–675.

STATUS: EVALUATION—NOT RELEVANT

54. Hazen PG. Skin cancer awareness programs: success of a statewide program of education and screening in Ohio. *Ohio Med.* 1989 Jun; 449–451.

STATUS: EVALUATION—NOT RELEVANT

55. Heneghan AM, Horwitz SM, Leventhal JM. Evaluating intensive family preservation programs: a methodological review. *Pediatrics.* 1996 Apr; 97(4): 535–542.

STATUS: REQUESTED REVIEW

56. Hingson R, McGovern T, Howland J, Heeren T, Winter M, Zakocs R. Reducing alcohol-impaired driving in Massachusetts: the Saving Lives Program. *Am J Public Health.* 1996 Jun; 86(6): 791–797.

STATUS: EVALUATION—RELEVANT

57. Howell E, Devaney B, McCormick M, Thiel K, Hill I. Reducing infant mortality through community-based initiatives: the Healthy Start Demonstration [abstract]. *AHSR FHSR Annu Meet Abstr Book.* 1994.

STATUS: NOT LOCATED

58. Hughes SL. Apples and oranges? A review of evaluations of community-based long-term care. *Health Serv Res.* 1985 Oct; 20(4): 461–488.

STATUS: REVIEW/POLICY/OPINION

59. Hunter JK, Crosby FE, Ventura MR, Warkentin L. A national survey to identify evaluation criteria for programs of health care for homeless. *Nurs Health Care.* 1991 Dec; 12(10): 536–542.

STATUS: METHODS

60. Indyk D, Belville R, Indyk LA. "Continuous quality improvement" approach to community-based program development: implications for understanding and meeting basic needs [abstract]. *AHSR FHSR Annu Meet Abstr Book.* 1994.

STATUS: NOT LOCATED

61. Kaltreider DL, St. Pierre TL. Beyond the schools: strategies for implementing successful drug prevention programs in community youth-serving organizations. *J Drug Educ.* 1995; 25(3): 223–237.

STATUS: REVIEW/POLICY/OPINION

62. Katzman MS, Smith KJ. Occupational health-promotion programs: evaluation efforts and measured cost savings. *Health Values.* 1989 Mar/Apr; 13(2): 3–10.

STATUS: REQUESTED REVIEW (METHODS)

63. Kegeles SM, Hays RB, Coates TJ. The Empowerment Project: a community-level HIV prevention intervention for young gay men [see comments]. *Am J Public Health.* 1996 Aug; 86(8): 1129–1136.

STATUS: EVALUATION—RELEVANT

64. Killen JD, Robinson TN, Telch MJ, Saylor KE, Maron DJ, Rich T, Bryson S. The Stanford Adolescent Heart Health Program. *Health Educ Q.* 1989 Summer; 16(2): 263–283.

STATUS: EVALUATION—RELEVANT

65. Kimel LS. Handwashing education can decrease illness absenteeism. *J Sch Nurs.* 1996 Apr.

STATUS: NOT LOCATED

66. Kishchuk N, O'Loughlin J, Paradis S, Masson P, Sacks-Silver G. Illuminating negative results in evaluation of smoking prevention programs. *J Sch Health.* 1990 Nov; 60(9): 448–451.

STATUS: METHODS

67. Kizer KW. Guidelines for community-based screening for chronic health conditions. *Am J Prev Med.* 1991 Mar–1991 Apr 30; 7(2): 117–120.

STATUS: REQUESTED REVIEW

68. Knudsen HC, Thornicroft G. Mental health service evaluation. <IM>New York : Cambridge University Press, 1996. *Studies in Social and Community Psychiatry.*

STATUS: REQUESTED REVIEW

69. Lando HA, Hellerstedt WL, Pirie PL, Fruetel J, Huttner P. Results of a long-term community smoking cessation contest. *Am J Health Promot.* 1991 Jul/Aug; 5(6): 420–425.

STATUS: EVALUATION—NOT RELEVANT

70. Laraque D, Barlow B, Durkin M, Heagarty M. Injury prevention in an urban setting: challenges and successes. *Bull NY Acad Med.* 1995 Summer; 72(1): 16–30.

STATUS: REVIEW/POLICY/OPINION

71. Liller KD, Smorynski A, McDermott RJ, Crane NB, Weibley RE. The MORE HEALTH bicycle safety project. *J Sch Health.* 1995 Mar.

STATUS: NOT LOCATED

72. Longo DR. The measurement of community benefit: issues, options, and questions for further research. *J Health Adm Educ.* 1994 Summer.

STATUS: NOT LOCATED

73. Marier AE. A health education program for migrant children. *Am J Public Health.* 1996 Apr; 86(4): 590–591.

STATUS: EVALUATION—NOT RELEVANT

74. Marshall E, Buckner E, Perkins J, Lowry J, Hyatt C, Campbell C, Helms D. Effects of a child abuse prevention unit in health classes in four schools. *J Community Health Nurs.* 1996; 13(2): 107–122.

STATUS: EVALUATION—NOT RELEVANT

75. Maslanka H, Lee J, Freudenberg N. An evaluation of community-based HIV services for women in New York State. *J Am Med Wom Assoc.* 1995 May/Aug; 50(3&4): 121–126.

STATUS: EVALUATION—NOT RELEVANT

76. Mayer JA, Kossman MK, Miller LC, Crooks CE, Slymen DJ, Lee CD Jr. Evaluation of a media-based mammography program. *Am J Prev Med.* 1992 Jan/Feb; 8(1): 23–29.

STATUS: EVALUATION—RELEVANT

77. McKeon T. Activity-based management: a tool to complement and quantify continuous quality improvement efforts. *J Nurs Care Qual.* 1996 Jan; 10(2): 17–24.

STATUS: REQUESTED REVIEW

78. McKinlay SM, Stone EJ, Zucker DM. Research design and analysis issues. *Health Educ Q.* 1989 Summer; 16(2): 307–313.

STATUS: METHODS

79. McLaughlin CP. Balancing collaboration and competition: the Kingsport, Tennessee experience. *Jt Comm J Qual Improv.* 1995 Nov; 21(11): 646–655.

STATUS: CASE STUDY

80. McLoughlin E, Vince CJ, Lee AM, Crawford JD. Project Burn Prevention: outcome and implications. *Am J Public Health.* 1982 Mar; 72(3): 241–247.

STATUS: EVALUATION—RELEVANT

81. McMeekin JC, Billings RW. A system that 'walks the talk'. Using improved community health status for CEO evaluation and compensation [interview by Karen Gardner]. *Trustee.* 1994 Apr; 6–9.

STATUS: REVIEW/POLICY/OPINION

82. Mersha T, Meredith J, McKinney, J. A grant rationing model for a health care system. *Socioecon Plann Sci.* 1987; 21(3): 159–165.

STATUS: REVIEW/POLICY/OPINION

83. Mittelmark MB, Hunt MK, Heath GW, Schmid TL. Realistic outcomes: lessons from community-based research and demonstration programs for the prevention of cardiovascular diseases. *J Public Health Policy.* 1993 Winter; 437–462.

STATUS: REVIEW/POLICY/OPINION

84. Mullen PD, Evans D, Forster J, Gottlieb NH, Kreuter M, Moon R, O'Rourke T, Strecher VJ. Settings as an important dimension in health education/promotion policy, programs, and research. *Health Educ Q.* 1995 Aug; 22(3): 329–345.

STATUS: REVIEW/POLICY/OPINION

85. Navarro AM, Senn KL, Kaplan RM, McNicholas L, Campo MC, Roppe B. Por La Vida intervention model for cancer prevention in Latinas. *J Natl Cancer Inst Monogr.* 1995.

STATUS: NOT LOCATED

86. Nelson S. How healthy is your school? guidelines for evaluating school health promotion. New York, NY: *NCHE Press*, 1986 printing.

STATUS: NOT LOCATED

87. O'Brien A, Anderson, C. Evaluation of the effectiveness of a community-based prenatal health education program. *Fam Community Health.* 1987 Aug; 10(2): 30–38.

STATUS: EVALUATION—RELEVANT

88. Pepe MC, Applebaum RA. Ohio's options for elders initiative: cutting corners or the cutting edge? *J Case Manag.* 1996 Spring.

STATUS: NOT LOCATED

89. Perry CL, Williams CL, Veblen-Mortenson S, Toomey TL, Komro KA, Anstine PS, McGovern PG, Finnegan JR, Forster JL, Wagenaar AC, Wolfson M. Project Northland: outcomes of a communitywide alcohol use prevention program during early adolescence. *Am J Public Health.* 1996 Jul; 86(7): 956–965.

STATUS: EVALUATION—RELEVANT

90. Roccella EJ, Horan MJ. The National High Blood Pressure Education Program: measuring progress and assessing its impact. *Health Psychol.* 1988; 7(Suppl.): 297–303.

STATUS: REVIEW/POLICY/OPINION

91. Rocheleau B. How do we measure the impact of intergovernmental programs? Some problems and examples from the health area. *J Health Polit Policy Law.* 1980 Winter; 605–618.

STATUS: REQUESTED REVIEW

92. Rogers J, Grower R, Supino P. Participant evaluation and cost of a community-based health promotion program for elders. *Public Health Rep.* 1992 Jul/Aug; 107(4): 417–426.

STATUS: EVALUATION—RELEVANT

93. Russell CK, Gregory DM, Wotton D, Mordoch E, Counts MM. ACTION: application and extension of the GENESIS community analysis model. *Public Health Nurs.* 1996 Jun; 13(3): 187–194.

STATUS: REQUESTED REVIEW (NEEDS ASSESSMENT)

94. Santelli JS, Celentano DD, Rozsenich C, Crump AD, Davis MV, Polacsek M, Augustyn M, Rolf J, McAlister AL, Burwell L. Interim outcomes for a community-based program to prevent perinatal HIV transmission. *AIDS Educ Prev.* 1995 Jun; 7(3): 210–220.

STATUS: EVALUATION—RELEVANT

95. Schulberg HC, Bromet E. Strategies for evaluating the outcome of community services for the chronically mentally ill. *Am J Psychiatry.* 1981 Jul; 138(7): 930–935.

STATUS: REVIEW/POLICY/OPINION

96. Schumacher JE, Siegal SH, Socol JC, Harkless S, Freeman K. Making evaluation work in a substance abuse treatment program for women with children: Olivia's House. *J Psychoactive Drugs*. 1996 Jan–Mar; 28(1): 73–83.

STATUS: EVALUATION—NOT RELEVANT

97. Shamai S, Coambs RB. The relative autonomy of schools and educational interventions for substance abuse prevention, sex education, and gender stereotyping. *Adolescence*. 1992 Winter; 27(108): 757–770.

STATUS: REVIEW/POLICY/OPINION

98. Shank JC, Erickson RA, Miller G. An assessment of the effect of "DOC talk" on school children in rural Iowa. *Fam Med*. 1987 Mar/Apr; 19(2): 129–132.

STATUS: EVALUATION—RELEVANT

99. Shea S, Basch CE, Wechsler H, Lantigua R. The Washington Heights-Inwood Healthy Heart Program: a 6-year report from a disadvantaged urban setting. *Am J Public Health*. 1996 Feb; 86(2): 166–171.

STATUS: EVALUATION—NOT RELEVANT

100. Sigelman C, Derenowski E, Woods T, Mukai T, Alfeld-Liro C, Durazo O, Maddock A. Mexican-American and Anglo-American children's responsiveness to a theory-centered AIDS education program. *Child Dev*. 1996 Apr; 67: 253–266.

STATUS: EVALUATION—RELEVANT

101. St. Pierre TL, Kaltreider DL, Mark MM, Aikin KJ. Drug prevention in a community setting: a longitudinal study of the relative effectiveness of a three-year primary prevention program in boys & girls clubs across the nation. *Am J Community Psychol.* 1992 Dec; 20(6): 673–706.

STATUS: EVALUATION—RELEVANT

102. Stolee P, Kessler L, Le Clair JK. A community development and outreach program in geriatric mental health: four years' experience. *J Am Geriatr Soc.* 1996 Mar.

STATUS: NOT LOCATED

103. Stone EJ. ACCESS: keystones for school health promotion. *J Sch Health.* 1990 Sep; 60(7): 298–300.

STATUS: REVIEW/POLICY/OPINION

104. Strobino D, O'Campo P, Schoendorf KC. A strategic framework for infant mortality reduction: implications for "Healthy Start." *Milbank Q.* 1995; 73(4): 507–533.

STATUS: REVIEW/POLICY/OPINION

105. Stryker J, Samuels SE, Smith MD. Condom availability in schools: the need for improved program evaluations. *Am J Public Health.* 1994 Dec; 84(12): 1901–1906.

STATUS: METHODS

106. Sweeney KA. School health screening: costs, benefits and alternatives. *Urban Health.* 1982 Nov/Dec; 46–49.

STATUS: REVIEW/POLICY/OPINION

107. Thacker SB, Koplan JP, Taylor WR, Hinman AR, Katz MF, Roper WL. Assessing prevention effectiveness using data to drive program decisions. *Public Health Rep.* 1994 Mar/Apr; 109(2): 187–194.

STATUS: REVIEW/POLICY/OPINION

108. Timko C. Physical characteristics of residential psychiatric and substance abuse programs: organizational determinants and patients outcomes. *Am J Community Psychol.* 1996 Feb; 24(1): 173–192.

STATUS: REVIEW/POLICY/OPINION

109. Von Korff M, Wickizer T, Maeser J, O'Leary P, Pearson D, Beery W. Community activation and health promotion: identification of key organizations. *Am J Health Promot.* 1992 Nov/Dec; 7(2): 110–117.

STATUS: REQUESTED REVIEW

110. Wechsler H, Weitzman ER. Community solutions to community problems—preventing adolescent alcohol use [editorial; comment]. *Am J Public Health.* 1996 Jul; 86(7): 923–925.

STATUS: REQUESTED REVIEW

111. Werch CE, Anzalone DM, Brokiewicz LM, Felker J, Carlson JM, Castellon-Vogel EA. An intervention for preventing alcohol use among inner city middle school students. *Arch Fam Med.* 1996 Mar; 5: 146–152.

STATUS: EVALUATION—RELEVANT

112. Werch CE, Young M, Clark M, Garrett C, Hooks S, Kersten C. Effects of a take-home drug prevention program on drug-related communication and beliefs of parents and children. *J Sch Health.* 1991 Oct; 61(8): 346–350.

STATUS: EVALUATION—RELEVANT

113. White J, Nezey IO. Project Wellness: a collaborative health promotion program for older adults. *Nursing Connections.* 1996 Spring.

STATUS: NOT LOCATED

114. Wholey JS. Perspective on evaluation from the U.S. Department of Health, Education, and Welfare. *Nurs Res.* 1980 Mar–Apr; 29(2): 109–112.

STATUS: REVIEW/POLICY/OPINION

115. Wilson-Brewer R. Comprehensive approaches to school-based violence prevention. *Health Aff (Millwood).* 1994 Fall; 167–170.

STATUS: REVIEW/POLICY/OPINION

116. Yancey AK, Walden L. Stimulating cancer screening among Latinas and African-American women. A community case study. *J Cancer Educ.* 1994.

STATUS: NOT LOCATED

117. Yawn BP, Lydick EG, Epstein R, Jacobsen SJ. Is school vision screening effective? *J Sch Health.* 1996 May; 66(5): 171–175.

STATUS: EVALUATION—NOT RELEVANT

118. Program evaluation: issues, strategies, and models. Washington, D.C.: *National Center for Clinical Infant Programs,* 1986 p. 20.

STATUS: NOT LOCATED

119. Price RH, Smith SS. A guide to evaluating prevention programs in mental health. Rockville, MD.: U.S. Department of Health and Human Services, Public Health Service, Alcohol, Drug Abuse, and Mental Health Administration, National Institute of Mental Health; Washington, D.C.: For sale by the Superintendent of Documents, U.S. G.P.O., 1985, vii, 135; ill. (Primary prevention publication series. 6, DHHS publication. no.(ADM) 85–1365.)

STATUS: NOT LOCATED

Table A.1

Inclusion and Exclusion Criteria for Literature Review

Inclusion Criteria
    Programs focused on people who are not patients or providers
    Randomized community trials
    Work-site health promotion (when work site is chosen as a locus of people, not a risk factor)
    School health
    Community-based programs related to substance abuse, mental health, long-term care[a]

Exclusion Criteria
    Not U.S.-based
    Program implemented pre-1975
    Randomized clinical trial
    Dental services
    Occupational health
    Emergency room, emergency response (e.g., train accidents), except for elder care personal emergency response systems
    Training programs unless effectiveness and evaluation specifically addressed
    Medical school or other professions, curricula development
    Medical school or other professions, training programs
    Managed care studies[a]
    Clinical public health projects[a]
    Quality improvement programs directed toward health professionals[a]

[a]Added after review of 1996 citations; see Chapter Three.

Table A.2

Summary of Published Evaluations Relevant to an Evidence-Based Approach to Decisionmaking for Community Health Interventions

	Author	Population	Setting	Health Problem	Outcome	Design
1.	Brink and Nader (1984)	Children	School	General health screen	Referrals, problems identified	Descriptive
2.	Bush et al. (1989)	Children	School	Cardiovascular risks	Blood pressure, cholesterol	RT[a] exp/cont[b]
3.	Campanelli et al. (1989)	Children	School	Alcohol	Knowledge, health perceptions	RT exp/cont
4.	Cohen et al. (1989)	Children	School	General health prevention (nutrition, blood pressure, smoking)	Knowledge, reported behaviors	Pre/post[c]
5.	Del Prete et al. (1993)	General population	General community/CBO[d]	Weight loss	Reported weight change	Pre/post
6.	Dielman et al. (1989)	Children	School	Alcohol	Reported behavior	RT exp/cont
7.	Dommeyer et al. (1989)	Young gay adults	College	AIDS	Attitudes/awareness	Pre/post
8.	Eisen et al. (1990)	Adolescents	School	Sexuality/contraception	Knowledge, reported behavior	Exp/cont
9.	Emery and Gatz (1990)	Elderly	CBO	Exercise/psychological health	Psychological well-being, cognitive function	RT exp/cont
10.	Flynn et al. (1994)	Children	School and general community	Smoking	Reported behavior	Exp/cont
11.	Fors et al. (1989)	Children and parents	School	Blood pressure	Knowledge, blood pressure, family interaction	RT exp/cont
12.	Gans et al. (1990)	Adolescents	School	Nutrition/cardiovascular risks	Cholesterol	Pre/post

Literature Identified 69

Table A.2 (continued)

Author	Population	Setting	Health Problem	Outcome	Design
13. Goeppinger et al. (1995)	Arthritis patients	CBO	Self-care	Self-care, pain, depression, psychological well-being	Pre/post
14. Guyer et al. (1989)	Children	General community	Injuries	Exposure, knowledge, reported behavior, injuries	Exp/cont
15. Hingson et al. (1996)	General population	General community	Alcohol/injuries	Reported behavior, alcohol MVA[e] fatalities	Exp/cont
16. Kegeles et al. (1996)	Young gay adults	Community	AIDS	Reported behavior, attitudes, exposure to intervention	RT exp/cont (1 community each arm)
17. Killen et al. (1989)	Adolescents	School	Cardiovascular risks	Knowledge, reported behavior, BMI,[f] HR,[g] skinfold	RT exp/cont
18. Marshall et al. (1996)	Adolescents	School	Child abuse	Parenting attitudes	Exp/cont
19. Mayer et al. (1992)	General community	General community	Breast cancer screening	Intention to obtain mammogram	Pre/post
20. McLoughlin et al. (1982)	General community	General community	Burn prevention	Knowledge, incidence/severity of burns	Exp/cont
21. MMWR (1996)	General community	General community	AIDS prevention	Exposure, reported behavior	Exp/cont multiple sites (1 RT site)
22. O'Brien and Anderson (1987)	Pregnant women	Community outreach clinics	Prenatal education	Hospital costs, OB complications	Exp/cont (very weak design)
23. Perry et al. (1996)	Adolescents	School/community	Alcohol	Reported behavior	RT exp/cont

70 Evidence-Based Decisionmaking for Community Health Programs

Table A.2 (continued)

	Author	Population	Setting	Health Problem	Outcome	Design
24.	Rogers et al. (1992)	Elderly	Community/CBO ambulatory care centers	General health screening/education + clinical examination	Perception of influence, satisfaction	Post survey of participants; descriptive
25.	Santelli et al. (1995)	General community	General community	AIDS prevention	Exposure, attitudes, reported behavior	Exp/cont
26.	Shank et al. (1987)	Adolescents	School	Prevention- STD/smoking/alcohol	Knowledge, reported behavior	Exp/cont (weak design)
27.	Sigelman et al. (1996)	Children	School	AIDS prevention	Knowledge, attitudes	Exp/cont (part random assignment)
28.	St. Pierre et al. (1992)	Children	CBO	Drug prevention	Knowledge, reported behavior	Exp/cont
29.	Werch et al. (1996)	Adolescents	School	Alcohol prevention (clinical)	Reported behavior, assessment results	RT exp/cont
30.	Werch et al. (1991)	Children and parents	School	Drug prevention	Reported behavior, knowledge, perceived impact	Exp/cont

aRT: randomized trial.
bexp/cont: experimental group vs. control group.
cpre/post: pre-intervention vs. post-intervention comparison only.
dCBO: community-based organization.
eMVA: motor vehicle accident.
fBMI: body mass index.
gHR: heart rate.

Appendix B
FOCUS GROUP PROTOCOL: FUNDERS

INTRODUCTION

Thank you for coming today. Before we get started, I would like to introduce myself and the other people working on this project. I'm Raynard Kington and this is Kathryn Pitkin and Catherine Jackson; we're from RAND. Kathryn Pitkin and I will be leading the discussion today, and Catherine Jackson will be taking notes and working the recording equipment. We also have with us today Arnold Tiemeyer from Main Line Health which is a partner organization in this project.

RAND is a nonprofit institution located in Santa Monica and Washington, D.C., and is dedicated to providing objective and scientifically sound public policy research. Main Line Health System is located in Philadelphia and is a network of nonprofit health care providers including the Jefferson Medical Center. We, RAND and Main Line, are partners in a project looking at ways community-based health programs are evaluated and funding decisions made.

The overall goal of this project is to explore the possibilities of developing an evidence-based approach to community health interventions decisionmaking. By an evidence-based approach, we mean a process by which decisions about which community-level health programs to implement are made based primarily on the strength of scientific evidence that a community-based approach or intervention will work. We also mean the rigorous application of scientific principles to assess, after implementing a program, whether it worked. By community-based, we mean those programs that might be conducted with local organizations at the "community level" that promote health or preventive health practices, such as parenting classes run by a community organization, radio announcements to discourage smoking, or church programs that promote the use of mammograms. We do not include in this category efforts that are normally implemented in a medical setting such as a hospital or a doctor's office.

In our discussion today, we are interested in learning how scientific evidence is brought to bear on decisions about funding and evaluation of your sponsored/funded programs, especially evidence on cost-effectiveness. We want to learn what key qualitative and quantitative indicators you use to assess cost-effectiveness, how you (and your organization) use such information when choosing between which programs to fund, and what types of monitoring systems you use or would like to see developed for implementation in programs.

GROUP PROCESS

We will ask you about how you and your organizations make decisions. We expect that some of you may work within quite formal criteria, whereas others of you may work with informal criteria. We hope that each of you in the group will speak up and contribute your ideas. Please try to speak one at a time, so we can hear from everyone. We hope not only that the discussion informs our project, but also that you find it interesting and stimulating. There may be times when I may interrupt the discussion and ask that we move to another topic or hear from someone else. I'll give you the "time out" signal when I need to do that. Please don't take it personally. It's just that time is short and we need to cover a lot of ground.

CONFIDENTIALITY

To have an exact record of what we discuss here today, we would like to tape this session. The focus group tapes will be listened to only by project staff. To encourage open discussion, we would like to keep the discussion anonymous. That is, we'll only use first names and not refer to our organizations or their sponsored programs by name. If you want to share that at the end of the session, that's OK. I should also mention that for the final report we will not attribute specific comments to any particular person or organization. We will be conducting several focus groups as well as structured telephone surveys, and will list participating individuals and organizations in the preface of the report. This will indicate to our funders and readers of the report that we have gotten input from a variety of organizations, while at the same time maintain confidentiality of participants' comments.

For now then, let's stay with first names only.

GROUP INTRODUCTIONS

I'd like to go around the table and ask each of you to introduce yourself. Please state your first name. <fill in this information on the seating chart>

Let's start with you . . . .

QUESTIONS

Types of Community-Based Health Programs

OK, let's start out by talking about the types of community-based health programs that your organizations fund.

If you don't mind, let's go around the table once more and each of you describe one typical or representative community-based program that your organization funds.

- What specific community or population does the program serve?
- What is the particular health issue being addressed?

Process of Funding Decisions

How does your organization make funding decisions regarding which programs to fund?

- Do you have competitive proposals?
- Does your Board make the decision?

- How do you choose between two (or more) program proposals?

Are your funding decisions influenced by proven efficacy or cost-effectiveness of the proposed program?

- Do you believe you have enough evidence about most programs to make a decision about likely efficacy or cost-effectiveness?
- Does such information exist and do you have ready access to it in a useful form?
- What type of information is missing? What information would you like to have to evaluate program effectiveness?
- Do you think your decisionmaking would improve with more information?
- Do you think that you have the scientific resources, either in-house or available to you in the form of advisory committees, to adequately judge the scientific evidence on the effectiveness of programs that you are considering funding?

Do you encourage potential fundees to provide in their application a summary of the best scientific evidence regarding the likely effectiveness of the programs under consideration?

Foundations often hear different priorities coming from the communities they serve. How do you go about balancing these various priorities?

- In what ways are your funding decisions influenced by the community?

How much influence or input do you provide prospective fundees regarding the types of programs your organization wants to fund?

- Do you essentially replicate the successes?
- Do you modify the failures and try again?

Process of Program Evaluation

How does your organization define program effectiveness?

How does your organization determine a successful program? Are successful programs always effective?

Does your organization routinely evaluate the effectiveness of the programs it funds?

How is this done?

- Program itself provides "production" statistics.
- Outside evaluation takes place.
- We conduct an evaluation.
- What types of inputs are normally part of the evaluation?
    — Client interviews.
    — Provider interviews.

Program Assistance

What does your organization do with programs that just aren't accomplishing the goals that were initially set?

- Does your organization provide technical assistance to struggling programs?
- Do you defund programs, or not renew their funding at the end of the contract cycle?

Wrap-Up

Is there anything else you would like to tell us that might help us understand how community-based health programs are funded and evaluated?

Close

On behalf of the project staff here today, I would like to thank you all for participating in this focus group today. The information and opinions you shared will help us better to understand the process through which funding organizations make decisions concerning the evaluation and funding of programs.

If any of you would like to see the final report, you can either give me your card or call me later. We'd be happy to share with you the results of our work.

Appendix C

TELEPHONE INTERVIEWS: SUGGESTED QUESTIONS FOR HEALTH SYSTEMS

1. Could you briefly describe your responsibilities, and how long you have held your current position?
2. a. Could you briefly describe what types of programs your organization has (conducts)?
   b. How much money does your organization dedicate annually to community-based health programs?
   c. On average, what is the size of the budget for a typical community-based health program that you sponsor?
   d. How many full- and part-time staff are involved in the decisionmaking process about which programs are implemented?
   e. How many full- and part-time staff in your organization are involved in monitoring or evaluating the projects that your organization does?
3. What kind of community-based programs is your organization currently conducting or sponsoring? How many of these programs do you have?
   a. What specific communities or populations do the programs serve?
   b. What are the particular health issues being addressed?

	Program	Community/Population	Health Issues Addressed
1.			
2			
3.			
4.			
5.			

4. Have you always done these types of programs, or have the program priorities of your organization changed? How have these changes occurred?

5. How does your organization make decisions regarding which community-based programs to do?

   a. Do you solicit competitive proposals from outside agencies?

   b. Does your Board make the decision about which programs to do?

   c. How do you choose between two (or more) programs?

   d. Are your decisions influenced by proven efficacy or cost-effectiveness of the proposed program?

6. How does your organization define program effectiveness?

7. How does your organization determine a successful program? Are successful programs always effective?

8. Does your organization routinely evaluate the effectiveness of the programs it sponsors? How is this done?

   — Program itself provides "production" statistics.

   — Outside evaluation takes place.

   — We conduct an evaluation.

   — What types of inputs are normally part of the evaluation?

      — Client interviews.

      — Provider interviews.

9. Do you believe you have enough evidence about most programs to make a decision about likely efficacy or cost-effectiveness?
10. Is it that the information doesn't exist or that you do not have ready access to it in a useful form?
11. What type of information is missing? What information would you like to have to evaluate program effectiveness?
12. Do you think your decisionmaking would improve with more information?
13. What does your organization do about programs that just aren't accomplishing the goals that were initially set?
    a. Does your organization provide or solicit technical assistance for struggling programs?
    b. Do you defund programs, or decide not to continue them?
14. Health systems often hear different priorities from the communities they serve. How do you go about balancing these various priorities? In what ways are your program decisions influenced by the communities you serve?
15. Is there anything else you would like to tell us that might help us understand how community-based health programs are funded and evaluated?

REFERENCES

Bero L, Rennie D. The Cochrane Collaboration: preparing, maintaining, and disseminating systematic reviews of the effects of health care. *JAMA.* 1995; 274(24):1935–1938.

Bero LA, Jadad AR. How consumers and policymakers can use systematic reviews for decision making. *Annals of Internal Medicine.* 1997; 126(1):37–42.

Brink SG, Nader PR. Comprehensive health screening in elementary schools: an outcome evaluation. *J Sch Health.* 1984 Feb; 54(2):75–78.

Bureau of Primary Health Care. *Models That Work: The 1995 Compendium of Innovative Primary Health Care Programs for Underserved and Vulnerable Populations.* U.S. Department of Health and Human Services, Public Health Service: Health Resources and Services Administration. U.S. Government Printing Office:1995. 404–882/21012

Carpinello SE, Newman DL, Jatulis LL. Health decision makers' perceptions of program evaluation. *Evaluation & the Health Professions.* 1992; 15(4):405–419.

Clancy CM, Kamerow DB. Evidence-based medicine meets cost-effectiveness analysis [editorial]. *JAMA.* 1996; 276:329–330.

Cook DJ, Mulrow CD, Haynes RB. Systematic reviews: synthesis of best evidence for clinical decisions. *Annals of Internal Medicine.* 1997; 126(5):376–380.

Del Prete L, English C, Caldwell M, Banspach SW, Lefebvre C. Three-year follow-up of Pawtucket Heart Health's community-based weight loss programs. *Am J Health Promot.* 1993 Jan/Feb; 7(3):182–187.

Dickersin KJ, Scherer R, Lefebvre C. Identifying relevant studies for systematic reviews. *Br Med J.* 1994; 309:1286–1291.

Doyle E, Smith CA, Hosokawa MC. A process evaluation of a community-based health promotion program for a minority target population. *Health Educ.* 1989 Dec; 20(5):61–64.

Emery CF, Gatz M. Psychological and cognitive effects of an exercise program for community-residing older adults. *Gerontologist.* 1990 Apr; 30(2):184–188.

Fishbein M. Great expectations, or do we ask too much from community-level interventions? [editorial]. *Am J Public Health.* 1996; 86(8):1075–1076.

Flynn BS, Worden JK, Secker-Walker RH, Pirie PL, Badger GJ, Carpenter JH, Geller BM. Mass media and school interventions for cigarette smoking prevention: effects 2 years after completion. *Am J Public Health.* 1994 Jul; 84(7):1148–1150.

Fortmann SP, Flora JA, Winkleby MA, Schooler C, Taylor CB, Farquhar JW. Community intervention trials: reflections on the Stanford Five-City Project experience. *Am J Epidemiol.* 1995; 142(6):576–585.

Goodman RM, Steckler A, Hoover S, Schwartz R. A critique of contemporary community health promotion approaches: based on a qualitative review of six programs in Maine. *Am J Health Promot.* 1993; 7(3):208–220.

Green SB. The eating patterns study—the importance of practical randomized trials in communities [editorial]. *Am J Public Health.* 1997; 87(4):541–543.

Green SB, Corle DK, Gail MH, Mark SD, Pee D, Freedman LS, Graubard BI, Lynn WR. Interplay between design and analysis for behavioral intervention trials with community as the unit of randomization. *Am J Epidemiol.* 1995; 142(6):587–593.

Guyatt GH, Sackett DL, Sinclair JC, Hayward R, Cook DJ, Cook RJ for the Evidence-Based Medicine Working Group. Users' guides to the medical literature. part IX: a method for grading health care recommendations. *JAMA.* 1995; 274(22):1800–1804.

Herman J. Second thoughts: the demise of the randomized controlled trial. *J Clinical Epidemiol.* 1995; 48(7):985–988.

Hingson R, McGovern T, Howland J, Heeren T, Winter M, Zakocs R. Reducing alcohol-impaired driving in Massachusetts: the Saving Lives Program. *Am J Public Health.* 1996 Jun; 86(6):791–797.

Horwitz RI. The dark side of evidence-based medicine [commentary]. *Cleveland Clinic Journal of Medicine.* 1996; 63(6):320–323.

Hunt DL, McKibbon KA. Locating and appraising systematic reviews. *Annals of Internal Medicine.* 1997; 126(7):532–538.

Kernick DP. Evidence-based medicine and treatment choices [letter]. *Lancet.* 1997; 349:570.

Killen JD, Robinson TN, Telch MJ, Saylor KE, Maron DJ, Rich T, Bryson S. The Stanford Adolescent Heart Health Program. *Health Educ Q.* 1989 Summer; 16(2):263–283.

Koepsell TD, Wagner EH, Cheadle AC, Patrick DL, Martin DC, Diehr PH, Perrin EB, Kristal AR, Allan-Andrilla CH, Dey LJ. Selected methodological issues in evaluating community-based health promotion and disease prevention programs. *Annual Review of Public Health.* 1992; 13:31–57

L'Abbe KA, Detsky AS, O'Rourke K. Meta-analysis in clinical research. *Annals of Internal Medicine.* 1987; 107(2):224–233.

Light RJ, Pillemer DB. *Summing Up the Science of Reviewing Research*, Cambridge, MA: Harvard University Press, 1984.

Mayer JA, Kossman MK, Miller LC, Crooks CE, Slymen DJ, Lee CD Jr. Evaluation of a media-based mammography program. *Am J Prev Med.* 1992 Jan/Feb; 8(1):23–29.

Maynard A. Evidence-based medicine: an incomplete method for informing treatment choices. *Lancet.* 1997a; 349:126–128.

Maynard A. Evidence-based medicine and treatment choices [letter]. *Lancet*. 1997b; 349:570–573.

McLoughlin E, Vince CJ, Lee AM, Crawford JD. Project Burn Prevention: outcome and implications. *Am J Public Health*. 1982 Mar; 72(3):241–247.

Mittlemark MB, Hunt MK, Heath GW, Schmid TL. Realistic outcomes: lessons from community-based research and demonstration programs for the prevention of cardiovascular diseases. *J Public Health Policy*. 1993 Winter:437–462.

Muir Gray JA. *Evidence-Based Healthcare: How to Make Health Policy and Management Decisions*, New York: Pearson Professional Ltd. 1997a.

Muir Gray JA. Evidence-based public health—what level of competence is required? *J Public Health Medicine*. 1997b; 19(1):65–68.

Mulrow CD, Cook DJ, Davidoff F. Systematic reviews: critical links in the great chain of evidence [editorial]. *Annals of Internal Medicine*. 1997; 126(5):389–391.

O'Brien A, Anderson C. Evaluation of the effectiveness of a community-based prenatal health education program. *Fam Community Health*. 1987 Aug; 10(2):30–38.

Pappas G, Queen S, Hadden W, Fisher G. The increasing disparity in mortality between socioeconomic groups in the United States, 1960 and 1986. *New England Journal of Medicine*. 1993; 329(2):103–109.

Rogers J, Grower R, Supino P. Participant evaluation and cost of a community-based health promotion program for elders. *Public Health Rep*. 1992 Jul/Aug; 107(4):417–426.

Rossi PH, Freeman HE. *Evaluation: A Systematic Approach*, 5th edition, Newbury Park, CA: Sage Publications, Inc. 1993.

Sackett DL, Rosenberg WMC. On the need for evidence-based medicine. *J Public Health Medicine*. 1995; 17(3):330–334.

Sackett DL, Rosenberg WMC, Muir Gray JA, Haynes RB, Richardson WS. Evidence-based medicine: what it is and what it isn't. *Br Med J.* 1996; 312:71–72.

Thacker SB, Koplan JP, Taylor WR, Hinman AR, Katz MF, Roper WL. Assessing prevention effectiveness using data to drive program decisions. *Public Health Rep.* 1994; 109(2):187–194.